THE LISTENING CHILD:
What Can Go Wrong

What all parents and teachers need to know
about the struggle to survive in today's
noisy classrooms

STEPHEN V. PRESCOD

Order this book online at www.trafford.com
or email orders@trafford.com

Most Trafford titles are also available at major online book retailers.

Every reasonable effort has been made to identify copyright holders. Stephen V. Prescod
would be pleased to have any errors or omissions brought to his attention.

Illustrated by Rita Lefebvre.

Printed in the United States of America.

ISBN: 978-1-4669-5163-1 (sc)
ISBN: 978-1-4669-5164-8 (e)

Library of Congress Control Number:2012916303

Trafford rev. 11/05/2013

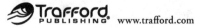 www.trafford.com

North America & international
toll-free: 1 888 232 4444 (USA & Canada)
fax: 812 355 4082

Dedication

To my one and only grandson Benjamin

SVP

Contents

PART I
Speech and Hearing Development

PART II
Beyond the Ear

PART III
MANAGEMENT

Foreword

Attention Deficiency Disorder (ADD), Central Auditory Processing Disorder (CAPD), problems related to information acquisition and retention, and a host of other learning and comprehension difficulties are all related to listening ability. Every day, teachers are faced with these problems in the classroom from kindergarten to high school. Parents, too, encounter these difficulties when they assist their children with assignments. These learning difficulties have an impact on the lives of many students.

The problem is that teachers who teach large classes, which now seem to be the norm in many educational jurisdictions, often detect these problems too late. Typically, children who experience learning problems give up in frustration or develop ways of dealing with their inability to listen effectively. They often try to cover up their deficiencies or compensate for them in various ways, for example, by faking knowledge or exhibiting aggressive behavior, both are symptomatic signs that students may be experiencing difficulties.

Teachers often have little time to spare for one-on-one remediation and are untrained or uninformed about the processing problems young listeners are experiencing in the noisy classroom. Many teachers at the elementary school level remain insensitive to the needs of these "underachieving" pupils as they are termed. In some cases, pupils with defective physical, emotional, or psychological capabilities are stigmatized and left behind to fend for themselves. The discovery of such problems often comes too late for the implementation of meaningful measures aimed at undoing the damage done to the child's self-esteem.

Dr. Stephen Prescod's book is an impressive comprehensive study of auditory processing disorders from which both a professional and a layperson can benefit. Dr. Prescod gives a thorough explanation of the physical mechanism associated with the child's auditory system and offers a carefully crafted explanation of the intricate physiological and perceptual processes that are involved in auditory communication (processes that communicators usually take for granted). He also goes on to explain the processes involved in how the child interprets and responds to information. Furthermore, he also explains how the child deciphers the myriad peripheral stimuli which impinge on the auditory system during his neuromaturational development as the child becomes increasingly aware of his environment.

Dr. Prescod reduces the technical language to a minimum so that the reader, whether a parent, teacher or academic, is able to understand very complex processes involved. He takes an incremental approach to the discussion of the problems encountered and encapsulates his findings in clear language. He then goes on to offer a number of practical suggestions and realistic solutions. Given his attention to detail and the well-explained methodology he proposes, the material in this book can be applied by any teacher, either trained or untrained, in dealing with the skills of effective listening and comprehension.

This book is an essential handbook for teachers of young children. Instructors at the elementary level informed by the material discussed in this book are more likely to interact with children in a sympathetic way and with a sharper focus on the process of listening. They will also be able to cooperate meaningfully with professional practitioners who offer remedial procedures. Knowledge of the potential problems and suggestions for their solutions will, I hope, dispose teachers to show more sensitivity to children who experience difficulty with auditory processing. No doubt, it will take the cooperation of parents, teachers, educators, and allied professionals if the child is to derive the maximum benefit from the implementation of solutions so clearly and methodically communicated in this work. I congratulate Dr. Prescod on his timely treatment of a subject that will remain topical as long as society considers it a priority to teach children to listen and to communicate effectively.

Leonard Adams, Ph.D. and Dip. Ed. in London University
Professor Emeritus, University of Guelph, Ontario, Canada

Preface

This book is a response to questions from hundreds of concerned parents and teachers as well as clinicians in the communication disorders field who are baffled by the behavior of certain children—children who, despite having normal hearing and intelligence, behave as though they were hearing-impaired and are seriously falling behind academically. These children have difficulty understanding what they are told. They seem to mishear speech and interpret information inaccurately which often leads to misunderstandings. They are socially isolated and at times labeled as daydreamers, slow, lazy, or unintelligent. Many of them behave as if they had a hearing impediment, yet hearing tests reveal that their hearing is normal. Still, since they persist in saying, "*What?*" or "*Huh?*" or "*I don't understand*," and at times, appear so lost when trying to comprehend simple instructions that teachers and parents are convinced they have a hearing problem. In fact, these children have what is known as a *central auditory processing disorder* (CAPD). This is a problem of impaired listening due to poor processing capabilities.

The ability to interpret information accurately is closely linked to auditory processing. In order for normal processing to occur, a number of cognitive auditory abilities must interact with fine-tuned precision at the cortical level with one objective, that is, to ascribe meaning to sound stimuli arriving at the brain. The efficient operation of these central abilities contributes to the normal auditory processing capabilities of the individual. How intelligently a child functions, depends on the speed and efficiency with which these central abilities are executed.

With normal auditory processing activity, the child listens intently as central auditory abilities interact with remarkable speed and efficiency to attribute meaning or symbolic significance to incoming stimuli. When these processes fail, and the central abilities perform with less than normal precision due to whatever prevailing conditions, the child is said to have a central auditory processing disorder or a performance deficiency in signal reception. This disorder or deficiency limits the child's ability to ascribe meaning to incoming stimuli so that he or she is neurologically impeded on expressive, receptive, and integrative levels from acquiring meaning. It is not surprising, then, that children affected, in this way have such great difficulty responding to simple commands and expressing themselves adequately through language. Indeed, no one really knows how they actually hear and attribute meaning to sound at all. It is clear, however, that with a defective auditory mechanism, it is bound to have a serious impact on a child's ability to learn.

Parents and teachers become increasingly frustrated when children are unable to attribute meaning to what they hear and are incapable of expressing formulated ideas appropriately in speech. In these children, something seems to intercept the steady flow of information from the ear to the brain and thus influence their ability to effectively translate sound into language. The brain is incapable of integrating, discriminating, and organizing input into meaningful patterns of information for academic purposes.

Such restrictive conditions predispose children to perform at an intellectually and socially subnormal level with reduced capacity to execute ordinary tasks compared to their normal processing peers. Teachers and parents are generally inclined to believe that these children have hearing problems or are unintelligent even though their hearing and intelligence may be professionally assessed as normal.

This book is intended to provide parents and teachers with some understanding of the conditions that cause these children to experience so much difficulty with auditory discrimination, memory tasks, attention span, and verbal skills. Though there is no reasonable explanation as to the etiology of the problem, the book takes a critical look at those factors—especially in the classroom—that tend to impede the learning process, restricting the child's ability to process information accurately and efficiently.

The book presents a theoretical approach to the problem of central auditory processing disorders or what is simply a dysfunction in signal reception. It examines the variables that affect listening and that subsequently interfere with learning. It suggests practical strategies for teachers who are dealing with children experiencing these perceptual difficulties on a daily basis.

The book stresses that a CAPD is not a single disorder but a matrix of disorders by briefly exploring how the hearing mechanism (receptive) part of hearing works and what can go wrong with it to affect the normal processing of information. It then looks at how the auditory processes involved in perceptive hearing work and what can also go wrong with these processes to influence the child's ability to manage the incoming information. Early learning signs are presented in both instances to alert the caregiver of potential hearing and listening problems that may have serious long-term consequences on the child's ability to learn.

It is the task of hearing and speech specialists, such as audiologists and speech-language pathologists, to identify the specific disorder, investigate its source, and then develop a deficit-specific management strategy tailored to the needs of the particular child. The main objective here is to help these children to overcome their deficiency so that they can realize their full potential and become functional and productive members of society. Once the problem has been identified, isolated, and treated, the child will learn to listen, to think and to process information as quickly and efficiently as any other normal listening child does.

The behavioral characteristics of children with CAPD are clearly delineated in the book, and it is hoped that with these guidelines, they will be more easily identifiable in the classroom so that remedial measures can be implemented at the earliest opportunity to address the problem. Most often, simple classroom strategies, when implemented appropriately, can produce remarkable strides in the retention and recall capabilities of the child for information that he or she might have otherwise misappropriated through poor listening skills that had been cultivated.

The book will appeal to a wide range of professionals, including academicians, researchers, special educators, teachers in special education, speech-language pathologists, audiologists, students, reading specialists, psychologists, physicians, the regular classroom teacher, and concerned parents.

Management is aimed at meeting the unusual needs of these children without labeling them as unintelligent or mentally deficient. How they learn depends to a large degree on how they are taught. But one thing is certain, neurologically, their brain is programmed for learning, and they learn successfully if taught correctly. To achieve this, they will require a smaller and more manageable learning space with reduction in noise levels for creative and productive thinking. If this can be achieved, with adequate staff and ample support systems in place, teacher, parent and above all student, would be sufficiently rewarded.

Stephen V. Prescod

About the Author

Stephen V. Prescod was Audiologist-in-chief for the Ministry of Health for the North Okanagon Health Unit in the province of British Columbia, Canada, before accepting a position with King Saud University, Riyadh, in the Kingdom of Saudi Arabia. Here he assisted in developing the undergraduate program in Speech Pathology and Audiology for students preparing for an advanced degree overseas in this field. He is a certified member of the American Speech-Language and Hearing Association(ASHLA) and the College of Audiologists and Speech Pathologists of Ontario(CASLPO).

Prescod's background includes an Assistantship at the State University of New York, a visiting Lecturer at Conestoga College, Ontario, an Associate Professor at Andrews University in Michigan and King Saud University in Riyadh, Saudi Arabia where he assisted in coordinating the Speech Pathology and Hearing Sciences program in the Department of Rehabilitation Sciences.

Prescod holds a double MA degree in Education and a MA in Clinical Audiology. He has a PhD from the State University of New York, in Diagnostic Audiology. He has contributed to several books and journals in the field of Education and Audiology. His latest book: "The Listening Child: What can go Wrong" addresses the problem of processing information under less than favorable learning condition within the classroom for children having processing problems. Central Auditory Processing Disorders is written for the first time in a language primarily suited for parents and teachers to understand, with recommended management strategies and protocols for these caregivers to utilize.

PART

I

Speech and Hearing Development

Introduction

How Processing Works
within the Child's Classroom
- An Overview

Auditory processing is an activity involving the auditory (hearing) system of the brain which is essential to the selection, separation, integration, clarification, storing and retrieval of all information received. All of these functions require a complex overlapping pattern of mental processes necessary to achieve understanding. The efficient operation of these processes is referred to as central auditory abilities- the end product of which is auditory perception.

In reality then, there is a distinction between the activity of hearing and that of listening. Simply put, hearing is an activity of the hearing end—organ mechanism, the cochlea. It's function is to receive sound stimuli from the ear, to be interpreted by the brain. Processing on the other hand, is the activity involving the decoding of neural impulses by the brain from the normal ear. This is referred to as the perceptive use of hearing. It is a cognitive activity, requiring special mental skills.

As long as the ear is functioning normally, it provides the basis for a complex ordering of skills so that processing can take place. It must be borne in mind however, that it is not the ear itself that does the possessing of information. The ear acts only as a conduit or conveyor of information to the brain. Therefore, it is possible for the child to have perfectly normal hearing, and yet fail to grasp anything the teacher is saying conceptually, since the brain may not be decoding stimuli it receives from the normal ear accurately. Thus the brain must decode the stimuli it receives with efficiency, in order to attribute meaning to what is heard by the normal ear.

This is what intelligent listening is all about. It is the means by which information is decoded from the ear to the brain accurately. It is the precise extraction of information form the auditory stimuli arriving at the brain level from the normal ear. When the brain is not decoding accurately, it is still possible for the child to hear sound such as the teacher's voice for example, and yet fail to make sense of what she is saying. Remember then, It is the ear that hears but it's the brain that attributes meaning to what is heard.

Under normal conditions, the brain is capable of processing information in microseconds. At any given moment in the classroom the child is bombarded by a host of sound stimuli. How intelligently a child performs within the classroom depends on the speed and efficiency with which auditory stimuli arriving at the brain is processed. When a child listens in the classroom, he is not in a state of passive cerebral inactivity, but is constantly assigning meaning to what the teacher is saying as long as the ear is functioning normally.

Once an acoustic signal reaches the normal ear (the teacher's voice for example), it has to be converted first from acoustic energy into electro-chemical energy before the child can make sense of what he or she hears. Once this transduction has taken place normally, it takes the brain only microseconds to attribute meaning to it. How does it accomplish this?

As we shall see later, the brain is in itself a complex storage and retrieval system which mandates that information be received, stored and organized in an orderly fashion if information is to be retrieved efficiently for future use. Thus, as an incoming signal reaches the brain, it compares incoming data from other sensory modalities, and from past similar learning experiences with the newly arriving information. Incoming stimuli are then organized into a latticework of interrelationships called concept formation, and at that point auditory perception begins. The brain is able to perform these functions in milliseconds as long as there is a built-in attention filtering device that assists in the processing of relevant information while filtering out that which is not relevant.

The child who processes information normally in the classroom, will have little difficulty assigning meaning to what the teacher is saying. However, the child with processing problems will, because he is not equipped with these excellent filtering capabilities of the normal processing child. He allows too much noise in the system thus both relevant and irrelevant stimuli easily overloads the circuitry of the brain. Furthermore, because of poor storage and retrieval capabilities of the brain, previous information has not been properly stored for future recall. This results in inadequate receptive, expressive and integrative function on the part of the child. He is therefore prone to perform at a significant disadvantage in the classroom. And since little thought has generally been given to his auditory needs and the conditions that best facilitate his learning, success cannot be assured.

Factors affecting auditory perception

Auditory perception is the brain's ability to decode, organize and encode incoming auditory stimuli in a meaningful and discriminative manner. It enables the child to make sense of what he hears. However there are many factors that may interfere with the normal influx of information to the brain of the child. These factors are likely to contribute to the delay of the transmission of impulses to the brain. This delay has the effect of interrupting the delicate fabric of interrelationships that make normal processing possible.

What are these factors that may intercept information to the brain? Factors such as noise interference, teacher/child placement—the greater the distance between teacher and child the more unfavorable the signal-to—noise ratio in the classroom, that is, as distance increases between teacher and child placement, the more distorted the signal reaching the child's ear from the teacher. Furthermore diseases such as ear infection, allergies, emotional instability of the child, teacher's *methodology and fear of the teacher etc., all of these and more are capable of contributing to the delay or blocking of transmission of impulses to the brain.*

When a child is forced to process information in an environment where those conflicting factors mentioned above are operating, they create a barrier to the effective transmission of information to the brain. When this is compounded by such afflictions as allergies and other upper respiratory diseases, it can only add to the difficulties in the classroom for the child. One day his hearing may be quite normal, and on another, his hearing may be inconsistent. The season, certain foods and environmental allergies all play a role in the way a child processes information from day to day in the classroom.

Finally, neural impulses may be altered or simply lost in the process of conversion or transduction from acoustic energy to electro-chemical energy. Thus gaps are created in the sequence of impulses available for decoding at brain level making it difficult for the child to make sense of what he hears. Many of these children are said to have central auditory perceptual problems.

Now how does all of this fit in with the learning process? First, let us take a look at what may be considered a normal processing model which incidentally is far simpler in concept than the more complex and intricate activity occurring at the brain level in reality. This simple model is just a model of convenience to help clarify a chain of complex events transpiring at brain level. This model is based on Semel (1970) model of auditory processing.[1] Responding to stimuli as has been pointed out earlier, all begins with a normal functional ear. The child's ear alerts him to sound in his environment. The sound within his environment requires him to constantly shift attention from foreground (primary signal of interest) to background(competing noise interference) within his environment in a matter of seconds. At this stage then, there is alertness, or awareness of something important in his environment, such as the teacher's voice.

Having been alerted to the teacher's voice, he must be capable enough in listening skills to separate the teacher's voice which he considers important, from the background interference which he considers interference. In order to do this effectively, he must first learn to focus on the signal (teacher's voice), then separate it from all other interference which is irrelevant. This is termed extractive listening, where the child pulls out from a background of irrelevant stimuli that which he considers relevant for processing. This is an extremely important listening skill. Extracting meaning from noise is an essential performance criteria children need in order to survive in the noisy classroom. It is a basic survival skill for everyday success in any classroom environment.

When a child cannot accomplish this skill, he misses large chunks of information that renders him incapable of remembering what has been said. Furthermore some children are easily confused when trying to accomplish more than one task simultaneously(multitasking) while trying to listen to the teacher. For instance, they may be trying to take notes from the teacher who they must track as she walks around the noisy room, while simultaneously try to decipher information from the chalkboard, while trying to make sense of what the teacher is saying. It is through the process of awareness that the normal processing child is able to "tune-in" and "tune-out" what he considers important and what he considers unimportant. When he unable to do this he misses vital portions of the message the teacher is delivering.

If that were all it would be difficult enough; but there are a number of other processes taking place at the same time as a part of awareness. For example, in order to achieve effective listening, he must also have a proper sense of spatial orientation to determine from which direction the sound is originating(localization). Also, through awareness, he must recognize that a signal has started, stopped, or even changed in some manner.

During this process the amount of information he receives for decoding depends on his ability to attend to the primary message without being confused with competing signals in his environment. This is where selective attention comes into play. He must be able to select the primary signal(the teacher's message), for processing, while suppressing or filtering out all other sources vying for his attention at the same time. Is it any wonder then that most children having auditory disorders are frequently confused with children having attention deficit disorder(ADD)?

The efferent system

Fortunately there is a system that aids the child in this process of selective listening. This system which is activated in the brain stem is known as the efferent system. When this system is intact and working optimally, a child makes selective judgment as to what is important for processing and what is not worth considering. This will be dealt with in more detail in a subsequent chapter.

Chapter 1

How We Hear

The Development of the Ear

The human ear is fully functional by the thirty-sixth week of gestation. By this time, the cochlea (end organ of hearing) portion of the bony labyrinth situated in the anterior aspects of the inner ear has become sophisticated in distinguishing sounds. The manner in which it analyzes sounds is somewhat restricted at this stage, however, due to lack of the maturation of the central auditory nervous system. But even then, there is evidence to suggest that "selective listening" of the fetus has already begun; that is, the fetus is already processing incoming stimuli and making distinctions between, for example, the mother's voice and other voices it hears (Kolata, 1984).

It is also believed that an unborn child, still protected in its mother's womb, is capable of responding to certain sounds long before it is born. Researchers have found that if a loudspeaker is placed near the mother's womb, a startled reflex to loud sounds can be elicited from the unborn child. It is here that the environmental enrichment begins to play an indispensable role in the child's capacity for discriminative and refined listening. *As a matter of fact, there is no period of parenthood with a more formative effect on development of the child's brain than the nine months of pregnancy leading to birth.*

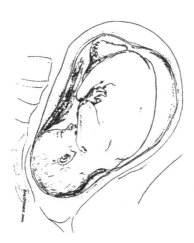

The unborn child

By the time, the baby is born the external ear (auricle) is formed and continues to develop until around age nine. The middle ear is also formed and effectively pneumatized (supplied with air pressure). The bones of the middle ear (ossicles) are already developed. The tympanic membrane (eardrum) changes relative position during the first two years of life while the inner ear is fully operative by the end of this two-year period. With a functional ear in place, the child is fully equipped to embark on the fascinating voyage of speech and language acquisition through the perception of sound. After birth, hearing enables a child to spin a web of language during his or her early growth and development. The development of listening skills starts at a very early age, and for a good reason, since it is by listening effectively through normal hearing processes that the child develops adequate speech *and language* function. That is because speech development is directly linked to hearing. A child who has difficulty hearing will naturally have difficulty acquiring appropriate speech patterns because all humans learn to speak by first hearing.

In order for the child to effectively process information he or she hears, both the *receptive* (decoding) and the *perceptive* (encoding aspects of hearing must be in perfect synchrony. Actually, the ear depends quite heavily on normal reception in hearing in order to transmit the correct signals it receives to the brain for cognitive processing.

As signals reach the brain and meaning is attributed to them, perceptive aspects of hearing or listening is at work. If anything is negatively affecting the receptive apparatus of hearing (the physical mechanism of the ear), the brain will be limited in its ability to process information it receives accurately. An infant who is developing proper listening skills, therefore, is not in a passive stage of development at all, but he or she adapts to the challenges of the listening environment and is involved in the profoundly dynamic and energetic undertaking, requiring the highest active capabilities (Friedlander, 1970).

The Hearing Mechanism

Technically, hearing actually takes place at the brain level and not at the ear level as is commonly assumed. The proper function of the ear is to change sound waves entering it into electrical signals (neural impulses) that the brain can understand. Sound waves enter the outer ear, pass through the auditory canal, and beat against a tightly stretched membrane called the eardrum (tympanic membrane) causing it to vibrate. The vibrations are picked up by three tiny bones (the tiniest bones of the body) housed in the pea-sized middle-ear cavity. These bones of the middle ear transmit the vibrations to the fluid-filled chamber of the inner ear via the stapes footplate.

Inside the fluid-filled chamber of the inner ear are thousands of specialized cells, each equipped with many microscopic hairs. These hair cells are immersed in the fluid that fills the inner ear chamber. They are set in motion whenever the fluid is disturbed. Stimulation of the hair cells by the disturbed fluid, in turn, generates electrical impulses that are sent on to the brain for decoding.

Hence, in order for a sound wave to reach the brain, the ear must first transform it into an appropriate medium that can be interpreted and understood by the brain. That appropriate medium is the *neural impulse*. It is the movement of the fluid in the inner ear that stimulates the attached cells to send a train of tiny neural impulses along the auditory nerve to the brain, where we eventually perceive them as sound. When any part of the hearing (receptive) mechanism cannot do its job efficiently, the transmission of sound to the brain is affected and the signals reaching the brain are not properly decoded. This results either in a hearing loss or a misrepresentation of the information received.

A delay in signal transmission to the brain caused by hearing loss or any other adverse listening condition in the environment, such as noise, causes the signal transmission to pick up distortion. The distortion can be created by a delay of just a few milliseconds in the temporal ordering of auditory symbols. The problem with the temporal ordering of language patterns brought on by even such a brief delay is that the delay causes the incoming impulses arriving at the brain to reach the brain out of phase or out of sequence with each other seriously restricting activity on the part of the child to attribute meaning to what he or she hears.

This has important implications for the function of the receptive processes of all children in general, but for those with central auditory processing disorders(*CAPD)* in particular. It is on the efficient transmission of stimuli to the brain that children depend for the acquisition of language, interpersonal communication, and learning. When this is affected, it creates processing difficulties forcing the child with CAPD to respond inconsistently to sound, causing him or her to be invariably misclassified as unintelligent, hearing-impaired, or mentally deficient.

Delayed signals arriving at the brain level out of phase are not clear, clean, or decipherable, and the brain cannot decode them efficiently. Under normal conditions, the brain processes information in milliseconds. But when the neural transmission to the brain has been altered in any way by unfavorable listening conditions such as noise, ear infection with middle ear fluid, emotional disturbance, or permanent hearing loss of the inner ear, the brain is unable to process incoming information with the speed and efficiency needed to generate understanding. When this occurs, the child then fails to maintain proper intellectual functioning known as useful auditory perceptual behavior. Indeed, any one of the hearing conditions listed below in this chapter can contribute to such auditory perceptual failure and seriously restrict comprehension.

Hearing Loss

Hearing loss is one of the limiting factors affecting how information is processed by the brain as well as how language is acquired by the child. It is one of the most serious and least recognized disabilities in children. The most critical years for detecting hearing loss are the preschool years and the lower elementary grade levels. Undetected and untreated hearing loss can have lasting effects on early speech and language development, learning, social growth, and the overall emotional stability of the child.

Even a minor hearing loss that is undetected can affect a child's academic and social development over time. Poor hearing is one of the most common undiagnosed problems responsible for children's learning difficulties. *It is not unusual for a child in such circumstances to be classified as mentally challenged, slow, inattentive, dull, and antisocial simply because he or she does not perform academically on par with his peers or participate in social activities like the rest of them.*

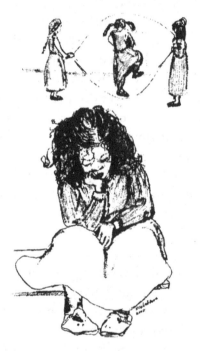

Hearing loss isolates the child

What is tragic is that children often conceal the harsh reality that they are unable to participate because of defective hearing. In Ontario, as many as one in four preschoolers has a communication disorder or significant language delay. At least, 6 percent of the total school population from junior kindergarten to grade 12 is affected (CASLPO, 2001).

- Studies has shown that if left undetected and untreated, even a mild hearing loss can reduce a child's academic achievement and cause educational retardation and deprivation
- cause the child to be falsely labeled as inattentive and speech delayed
- increase behavioral problems, causing social isolation, and accompanying psychological and emotional disturbance
- cause permanent hearing loss if untreated for an extended period of time.

Children with early language-processing difficulties are ten times more likely to have associated behavioral problems than those without such difficulties. It has been shown that 60 percent of children with behavioral disorders have significant language problems and a further 75 percent to 80 percent of students with learning disabilities have related language problems (OSLA, 1996). Hearing loss is crucially linked to impaired language development. Since speech develops as a direct consequence of hearing, children with hearing impairment experience difficulty developing normal speech along with delays in other aspects of academic functioning. The most likely results include the following:

- Academic delays especially in reading and mathematical concept formation.
- A 43 percent drop-out rate compared to 23 percent in nonimpaired children.
- Consistent rating and labeling of children with language disorders as nonintelligent and academically slow.
- Falling behind in school—children with mild to moderate hearing losses perform 1 to 4 grades behind peers with normal hearing.
- Low educational levels (children with severe to profound hearing losses generally achieve no higher than third or fourth grade level, unless early and appropriate intervention have been implemented).

Prolonged absence of normal stimulation to the cochlea because of ear infection or hearing loss can and does produce an altered abnormal physiological response to auditory signals reaching the brain for processing. The prolonged absence of normal stimulation creates what is known as *auditory sensory deprivation*. Auditory sensory deprivation alters the quality of the signal reaching the brain for processing as action potentials (neural discharges) to the brain are blocked. A deprivation of input means that the neurological processes by which this child learns will be altered.

A defective hearing apparatus will most certainly distort those signals that are changed into neural impulses for the brain to use. This impedes learning because the information conveyed through the peripheral mechanism, namely, the ears, is disrupted by hearing loss, and the central auditory nervous system is not able to use the information received, since it is highly distorted from the impaired ear.

When signals or neural impulses are distorted, the brain is forced to process distorted signals, and it is these signals that are reinforced by the child over and over again, becoming established patterns of communicative behavior, until the child, through proper training and therapy, is in a position to correctly display behaviors that are acceptable. Therefore, the earlier a hearing loss is detected and treated, the better the chances that the treatment will be effective and that associated problems in communication will be less severe.

Some children are born with defective hearing while others lose hearing abilities because of an illness or accident. In either case, the earlier the diagnosis and treatment, the better the prognosis for successful communication and the more the child can rely on the auditory channel for efficient transmission of information to the brain. It is for this reason that the Joint Committee on Infant Hearing, 1990 *Position Statement* endorsed the goal of universal detection of infants with hearing loss as early as possible. It recommends that all infants with hearing loss be identified before three months of age and receive intervention at least by six months of age.

Since it has been shown that hearing loss has significant implications for the normal development of speech perception, cognitive, psychosocial skills, and overall academic achievement early identification cannot be overemphasized. The design of comprehensive intervention strategies that address the overall development of not merely language but the academic, psychosocial, and developmental communicative experience of the child is of prime importance (Johnson, 2001).

Types of Hearing Loss

Let us now examine some of the things that can go wrong with the receptive apparatus of hearing and the ways in which they may influence the child's ability to process information normally. There are four different types of hearing conditions that may result from a malfunctioning hearing apparatus and, therefore, limit the scope of decoding capabilities of the brain— conductive hearing loss, sensorineural hearing loss, mixed hearing loss, and central hearing loss (which will be dealt with separately in Part II of this book). Any or a mixture of these conditions can affect the way a child's brain processes information.

Conductive Loss

Outer Ear

A conductive hearing loss is a loss of hearing caused by blockage of sound waves reaching the inner ear. This blockage reduced mechanical movement in the outer and middle ear, causing a conductive hearing loss. In most cases, early detection and treatment of a conductive hearing loss enable prevention of further impairment of the hearing apparatus. Transmission of sound waves may be blocked by damage or malformation of outer and middle ear structures. It is important to note that as long as this occurs sound will not be transmitted efficiently to the brain, and all sound entering the ear will be weaker, delayed, and distorted to some degree as it arrives at the brain for processing.

Occasionally, the outer ear may be incompletely formed, resulting in partial or complete blockage. This condition can be treated by surgical means by simply widening the existing canal or by opening a new canal if the passageway is completely blocked. In any event, a hearing loss usually results from conditions of this kind until the situation can be surgically treated.

Another condition that may affect the outer ear canal is the accumulation of wax, which prevents effective sound transmission from reaching the eardrum. Periodic removal of wax by a qualified practitioner will solve this problem by professionally removing the wax from the ear.

Finally, the outer ear may be infected by disease causing redness, irritation, and rawness of the skin tissues that line the canal walls of the ear. This condition is referred to as *external otitis* and is usually amenable to medication

Middle Ear

The middle ear (or tympanic cavity as it is called) is an air-filled cavity or chamber. Air pressure is necessary for the general good health of the middle ear and for its proper function. The middle ear consists of the eustachian tube, mastoid antrum, and mastoid air cells. They are jointed together to form a continuous air space. It is the eustachian tube that constantly maintains the equilibrium between the middle air pressure and the external air pressure.

Allergies, colds, and ear, nose, and throat infections occasionally cause the eustachian tube to close, thus upsetting the delicate equilibrium in pressure balance between the middle ear and external ear and causing fluid to build up in the middle ear space. The accumulation of fluid is called *serous otitis media (SOM)*. Serous otitis media usually follows a cold and also occurs as the residual condition of *acute otitis media*, particularly when antibiotic therapy has been ineffective.

The eustachian tube connects the middle ear cavity with the back of the throat. The upper end of the tube is normally kept open while the lower end is normally closed or collapsed because it is surrounded by soft tissue. Childhood diseases, such as upper respiratory and subsequent middle ear infection and closure of the eustachian tubes by enlarged adenoids, are among the known causes of middle ear problems that can result in conductive hearing loss. In the case of enlarged adenoids, for example, the eustachian tube opening may become blocked, leading to infection of the middle ear cavity. When tonsils and adenoids are infected in this manner, a physician decides what course of action or treatment would be most effective in resolving the problem.

The pus that forms and settles in the middle ear space as a result of diseased condition, occasionally, causes discomfort and hearing loss. If promptly treated medically with antibiotics, this condition is likely to pass. If left untreated, serous otitis media, with its accumulated middle ear fluid, can eventually rupture the eardrum. This mastoid bone marrow and tissue may also become infected in the process, causing a condition known as *mastoiditis*. These conditions must be treated quickly and effectively with medication, or in some cases, by surgery to avoid serious complications of the middle ear and other parts of the auditory system.

Another condition that can affect middle ear function and result in hearing loss is a *ruptured or perforated eardrum* caused by factors such as extreme air pressure changes in the external ear canal, pressure from accumulated middle ear fluid against the drum, or accidental injury. Traumatic insult to the eardrum, for example, can also cause dislocation of the tiny bones of the middle ear, resulting in hearing loss.

Severe trauma can extend to the inner ear as well, resulting in permanent damages and loss of hearing. While a ruptured eardrum may heal naturally, if left unattended, it leaves a thickened scar, resulting in mild hearing loss. In more severe cases, surgery may be required to improve hearing. In the case of total absence of an eardrum, for example, reconstructive surgery may be necessary to improve hearing function.

Finally, the three tiny bones of the middle ear may become immobilized by a condition called *otosclerosis*. Otosclerosis is caused by deposits between the stapes bone of the middle ear and the oval window of the inner ear. These deposits eventually restrict movement or immobilizes the middle ear bone's lever action, causing head noise (tinnitus) and significant hearing loss. Surgery known as a *stapedectomy* is usually required in such cases to improve middle ear function.

Persistent conductive hearing loss, which may result from the above conditions, interferes with the educational performance of children in their formative years and must be detected and treated early and effectively to avoid unnecessary long-term developmental consequences for the child's social and academic performance. With middle ear infection, known as otitis media, the persistent "runny nose," watery eyes, mouth breathing, and snoring resulting from an unbroken cycle of ear infection create a prolonged absence of normal stimulation to the end organ of hearing. As mentioned earlier, if continued unchecked, this condition will alter the physiological response of the brain to sound, restricting its capacity to process information efficiently, and seriously impeding the child's ability to learn.

Sensorineural Loss

Inner Ear

Sensorineural or inner ear hearing losses are for the most part not preventable or correctable by medical or surgical means. However, (re)habilitative measures when carefully implemented allow children to take their normal place in society as functional and productive individuals. Sensorineural hearing loss may be caused by damage to the delicate structures of the inner ear or the auditory nerve along with the sensitive nerve mechanism that is responsible for converting mechanical energy into neural impulses. These conditions can result in permanent sensorineural hearing loss. Some causes of sensorineural hearing loss in children are pregnancy related. These are the following:

- *Rubella (German measles): there is a 14 percent chance of the unborn child having hearing loss if the mother contracts the disease during early pregnancy*

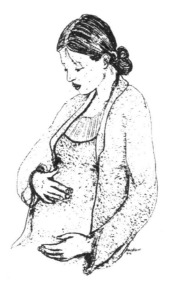

Pregnant mother with Rubella (German measles)

- RH blood type incompatibility—this is now preventable by serum injection
- birth injury
- premature birth—chances of hearing loss are greatly increased
- birth defects from hereditary causes
- childhood diseases occurring with high fever, like scarlet fever, whooping cough, mumps, meningitis, and influenza

- toxic effects of drugs

As far as the toxic effects of drugs are concerned, it is important to note that congenital as well as acquired hearing loss can occur from ototoxicity if taken by pregnant women without proper medical supervision. Most of the critical events in the development of the human ear take place during the four to five weeks after conception. Therefore, during this critical period if a mother catches an infection or take any ototoxic drugs without medical supervision, the developing child can be at risk for permanent damage to hearing. All of the above conditions have the potential to interfere with the child's ability to hear and to develop normal speech and language skills as well as proper processing capabilities.

It is often difficult for caregivers to detect early signs of hearing impairment in their children. However, if a child is not trying to talk by age one or seems insensitive to sound at any age, this is cause for concern. When a hearing loss has been uncovered, its progress should be monitored for habilitative purposes. In the event the hearing appears to be getting progressively worse, a more extensive physical examination is warranted. Caregivers, audiologists, and otologists must be aware of the subtleties of genetic deafness, which is known to cause rapid or gradual deterioration of hearing.

When sensorineural hearing loss is detected and treated early, the chances for communication are good. The likelihood of the child developing proper communication skills with the use of advanced technology in available educational and personal amplification systems is very high. With a properly fitting hearing aid, results are often spectacular. When the condition is detected early enough, learning improves, vocalization is increased, and the child becomes more alert, cooperative, and increasingly able to interact with his or her environment.

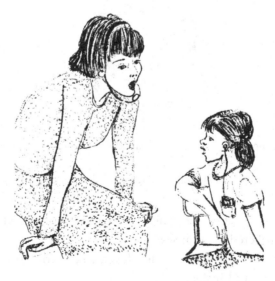

Educational amplification facilitates learning

Mixed Hearing Loss

Some hearing losses involve both the conductive and sensorineural mechanisms. In other words, both the outer and /or middle ear are involved along with the inner ear. These are called *mixed* losses. Again, early detection and treatment is the key to effective management and to minimizing the severity of problems in the long run. When a conductive loss appears superimposed on a sensorineural hearing loss producing a subtle type of hearing difficulty, it requires the skill of an audiologist to detect it; otherwise, the superimposed loss may go undetected. It is, therefore, necessary for children having sensorineural hearing losses to go for regular hearing checks by an audiologist to assure that a conductive loss is not superimposed on the already existing sensorineural hearing loss.

There is a fourth kind of hearing deficiency which shall be dealt with at length in the second part of this book; the central auditory processing deficiency (CAPD) that occurs when the hearing centers of the brain receive signal information incorrectly. Children with this disorder do hear, but may have difficulty understanding what they hear.

Chapter 2

The Child's Speech and Hearing Development

To determine whether the child's hearing and speech processes are developing normally, it is necessary to compare these processes to what may be considered a normal developmental model, in which, behaviors fit neatly into a predictable pattern. It is, therefore, important to know how the communication of normal infants evolves and what constitutes the developmental norms for auditory, language, and speech acquisition.

Generally speaking, normal hearing children develop language naturally as long as they are placed in the proper environment to do so. Since the verbal symbols associated with language emerge spontaneously, principally because of normal hearing—which provides the primary means through which hearing children develop and use language—when certain stages of development are either delayed or missed, caregivers and professionals should investigate the cause(s) as soon as possible and intervene where necessary with remedial measures. Early intervention allows the child to take advantage of the critical period of language development, bringing about effective and permanent change in the evolution of appropriate patterns of communication.

According to research, language is a human instinct based on genetic instructions and on the maturing of language centers in the child's brain (Pinker, 1994). But all of this presupposes that the basic anatomical, neurological, and psychological processes are intact, that is, there is a normal brain, adequate hearing, normal peripheral anatomical structures used in speech, as well as a stimulating environment (Karlin, 1958).

Normal children have a built-in feedback system or a monitoring capability that works very effectively toward the gradual acquisition of speech and language function. As children compare their own verbal production with incoming verbal stimuli, they progressively match them with what they hear, to the point where these productions are refined so that they eventually replicate what they hear. In this way, children progressively move closer and closer toward an acceptable standard of production. But it is important to remember that children do not only hear the vocalization of others, but they also hear and monitor themselves constantly, as long as the hearing apparatus is functioning normally. When it is, children are, therefore, able to progressively refine their vocalization activities over time.

There is an extraordinary period of development in the communication process starting very early in the child's life. In fact, this development is so rapid and miraculous that it is often regarded as an automatic, maturational process. Some place this period between eighteen and thirty-six months after birth; others argue that it is actually the formative years between birth and four years of age that constitutes the optimum period for fostering speech and language development. Yet others contend that the optimum period is between birth and three years of age and that the "readiness to speak" period is between twelve and eighteen months. Whatever the precise time frame, it is during the early formative years that the child's listening skills must be refined to their maximum through increased levels of environmental stimulation, which in turn enhances the development of the vitality of the cortex.

Furthermore, the more the child is exposed to language in the environment and provided with the opportunity to use it, the more abundantly the neural circuits are pruned into a left hemisphere pattern of specialization for language. Therefore, the more exposure to verbal input exists, the more the left hemisphere specializes in receiving and producing words and the thicker the speech areas of the cerebral cortex becomes.

Not all children will follow the developmental schedule for communication as precisely as it is outlined below since children differ greatly in abilities and growth characteristics. Some children will follow a slower maturational schedule than others and reach landmarks of development later than their counterparts. We do know, however, that children have an innate capacity for developing language skills, given appropriate exposure to an adequate sample of language at an early age. *Therefore, a child, who is healthy and yet shows no consistent response to sound and who is not developing speech according to the developmental model, is most certainly a cause for concern.*

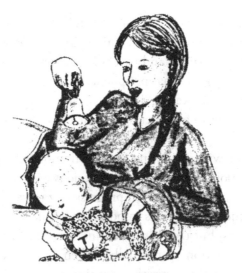

The silent child

When a child is experiencing difficulty hearing sounds and hearing differences in sounds, he or she does not develop speech or language on schedule. Understanding what is heard and attributing meaning to it is difficult if not impossible. However, concern here must be tempered with caution, and we should not leap to premature conclusions, regarding the status of the child's communication development. Individual differences occur and must be taken into account when interpreting what may be regarded as normal compared to what may be regarded as abnormal communication development. All we can say is that an appropriate response to sound is missing and professional investigation is warranted.

At any rate, suspicion of communication delay would warrant professional consultation with a speech-language pathologist and an audiologist so that intervention could be started at the earliest opportunity if problems are identified. In the event of identification, it would be unfortunate to defer immediate intervention until later in the child's development. The longer the delay, the poorer the prognosis for the child's overall success. Therefore, regardless of whether the purpose is prevention or remediation, intervention should start as early as possible after communication problems are identified.

When hearing problems of significance are present, the child will not develop speech and language at the normal rate. As a part of the habilitative process, parents are encouraged to get involved with intense speech and language stimulation at the earliest opportunity. Caregivers should engage as much as possible with the child, encouraging appropriate language response. Such activities stimulate listening as caregivers persistently talk and communicate with the child to generate an awareness of correct sounds and speech patterns.

Encouraging the child to speak at every opportunity, engaging him or her in meaningful play activity, and rewarding word-appropriate response together with praise and reinforcement when the child responds successfully—all of this not only improve the quality of the time spent together but also develop appropriate listening and language function. Even a child with severe hearing impairment can still recognize a few simple lip movements at five to eight months of age and should be encouraged to communicate.

A child's ability to use language is closely related to his ability to process speech through the ear (Pinheiro, 1977). When acquiring language skills, the child first analyzes the sounds he hears before being able to speak. These sounds later develop into words and phrases, which are the cornerstone of language. It is during these early developmental years that caregivers must interact with children and encourage them to become aware of different types of sounds and their associated meanings until children learn to respond appropriately to sounds that are meaningful.

At the same time, it is equally important to be aware of the warning signs when these behaviors are delayed or absent. Observation of communication development during infancy, reveal the presence or absence of sensory and motor difficulties the child may be encountering.

Early warning signs that should alert parents to hearing difficulties in older children are as follows:

- The child seems to favor one ear when listening.
- The child fails to respond when questioned and seems to hear only incomplete conversation and must have things constantly repeated
- The child is listless and inattentive.
- The child listens to radio and TV at very loud levels in spite of the high volume, he or she sits right up to the TV to hear.
- The child complains of frequent earaches or ringing and discomfort of the ear
- The child asks to speak up or complains of people mumbling.
- The child tends to watch lips of the speaker for understanding.
- The child talks unreasonably loud with peculiar voice quality.
- The child has defective speech.
- The child often misunderstands what people are saying.
- The child has poor oral reading ability and tends to run words together.
- The child complains frequently of head noise, earaches, and discharging ears and may hold head in a peculiar position with listening.

The Speech and Hearing Developmental Model

The basic information about normal auditory infant aural—oral development is given below. Again, these are simply guidelines as there is a range of individual difference to consider when interpreting behaviors of this kind. However, if any one of these indicators suggests a problem, professional investigation is warranted.

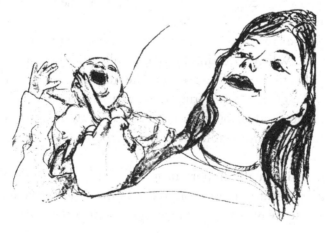

The birth cry

Birth to Three Months

From the time babies enter the world, they have an insatiable desire to communicate. The baby's first utterance is the "birth cry." The birth cry announces that the baby is now ready to assume his or her position as an integral part of society. It also indicates that his or her neurological and physiological processes as well as motor development are intact. Newborns are well on the way to further development and learning has already begun. The partnership between caregiver and child has begun as well. Within weeks, the child will be able to vocalize a variety of sounds and use them effectively to have this or her needs fulfilled.

The infant's cry modifies over time and rapidly gives way to a repertoire of sounds and vocalizations that carry with it significant implications. As time passes, a discerning mother will notice distinctive changes in the character of the infant's utterances. There is a qualitative difference between the cry of pain and the cry of hunger. Similarly, vocalization for pleasure is distinctively different from that for attention. At this stage, infants are effectively using various types of utterances to express their needs and desires. From then on, they are intently preoccupied with sound and with responding to it as hearing and vision interact to reinforce visual symbols during the early weeks of life. But it is primarily through hearing that verbal language emerges during these early months. Infants become more and more secure in monitoring the environment in which they live and have an increased capacity to make selective responses to fine auditory signal differences. It is critical at this period that they are not left to cry on indefinitely without having their needs satisfied.

In the first months following birth, babies listen intently to the sound of mother's voice and the sound of their own voice as well as to the sounds in their immediate environment. In fact, as they become aware of their own voice—how it sounds and what capabilities it has—this voice takes precedence in interest over all other sounds in the environment. At this early stage of development, caregivers should imitate the sounds babies make and encourage them to make even more. The first noncrying speech sounds babies use are vowels with about four different vowels heard during the first two months, and one new vowel should be added every two months for the first year.

Soon children start using their own voice to express feelings of pleasure, anger, or sadness. For example, when a toy is taken away or some activity is forbidden, they express anger. On such occasions, it is important _to_ let them know that you understand what they are experiencing. When they are happy, let them know what good children they are, and when they are sad, show them you emphathize.

Warning Signals

Within three months of age, an infant should

- be soothed by the mother's voice
- use different cries to express different needs
- attend to familiar voices
- exhibit the *startle reflex* when surprised

The first warning sign of concern is that baby pays no attention to the mother's face. Within the first four weeks of age, babies normally watch mother's face intently as she speaks to them. If the baby is not attentive to the mother as she speaks or if loud and strange sounds do not startle, frighten, or amuse him or her, or the baby does not notice the sound of footsteps approaching the crib or does not respond to the mother's voice before seeing her, something could be wrong. All of these signs must be taken seriously and should be investigated at the earliest opportunity.

The startle reflex is generalized body movement of the child to moderately loud sound, such as a handclap a meter or two away or sudden noises in the immediate environment. If the baby is not startled by these, the startle reflex is absent. This generalized response starts to fade away at around twelve weeks of age. It becomes more inhibited as the central mechanism of the auditory nervous system matures and takes over control of auditory responses. By sixteen to twenty weeks, the "startle reflex" fades away entirely and is replaced by children turning their head toward the source of sound. *The absence of any generalized body movement involving more than one limb and accompanied by some form of eye movement in the presence of a loud sudden noise is cause for concern.* So is a situation when the child is not quieted by the mother's voice.

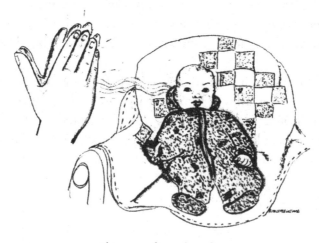

Absence of startle reflex

Four to Seven Months

By the fourth to sixth month, the behaviors referred to earlier are beginning to crystallize. Children increasingly refine their own sounds with spontaneous cooing. Babbling—a series of syllabic repetitions—is now a frequent part of children's developing vocabulary, especially when they are alone. This form of behavior is distinctly human since only human babies babble and is, therefore, the first expressive human act in terms of communication in which the child engages. Babbling signals that physiological and psychological processes are intact and developing normally. Babies who coo and babble regularly are the ones who make the most rapid progress in the development of speech.

During this period, children

- anticipate sounds associated with feeding
- deliberately turn head to voices and search for the source with eye movement
- hold their head erect
- continue to chuckle and gurgle
- laugh aloud (laughter is socially oriented at this time and is stimulated by affectionate play with other persons)
- experience a surge in motor development, accompanied by incessant cooing and babbling, as well as use the sounds heard in the environment.

In order to babble, children must learn to coordinate the musculature of articulation, phonation, and respiration, which is so vital to normal speech development. It is during this stage that a variety of syllables are heard. Articulation development parallels his motor development, and both become more refined as time goes by. Children enjoy vocalizing to a mirror image. They respond meaningfully to expressions of anger or pleasure and are now more responsible to soft meaningful sounds than to loud environmental sounds, which seem of little interest to them. They are soothed by the sweet lullaby of the mother's voice and fall asleep upon hearing it.

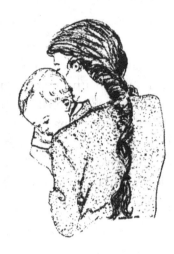

The baby is soothed by the mother's voice.

Warning Signs

The absence of babble at this stage is cause for concern. Deaf children do not babble, neither do autistic children. Why don't they babble? Because, in both instances, they are marked disturbances in either their physiological or their psychological development. Deaf children generally have a profound hearing loss and, therefore, cannot utilize sound meaningfully for communicative purposes. Autistic child have marked psychological disturbances that limit meaningful contact and communication.

The time at which sound becomes meaningful coincides with the ability to localize familiar sound, especially the human voice. Therefore, absence of a sharp turn of the head or any other obvious change of activity in response to loud, sudden sounds in the environment at this stage may be a sign of auditory dysfunction. If the child does not turn his head to localize sound or does not react to familiar sounds in the environment such as the barking of the dog, the meowing of the cat, the ringing of the doorbell or telephone, or the calling of his or her name, appropriate professionals should be consulted for advice.

Furthermore, if the child does not repeat sounds he or she makes or hears others make, at this stage of development, this also signals a potential problem. Children who show no interest in familiar meaningful sounds or uses no vocalization or babbling in relation to their environment may be experiencing auditory difficulties that require professional assistance.

Eight to Twelve Months

At this stage, two-syllable repetitive babbling has begun (children repeat combinations of two or more different sounds) and inflections in vocalization increasingly resemble speech. There are marked rhythm patterns in vocalization. Children respond to their own babbling, but the babbling is being modified constantly as they receive more auditory impressions and imitate parents. By imitation, they are establishing the vital link between hearing and speech, and the sounds are becoming closer to the target sounds that characterize the speech of others around them. There are more consonant sounds at this stage as children prepare to use their first word.

As communication develops, children become familiar with the auditory sensations and motor adjustments necessary to make and change sounds. They proceed from differential babbling to the imitation of linguistic and nonlinguistic sounds they hear. This process must be encouraged by caregivers, who should match the children's efforts by modeling new structures for him to imitate.

By now, children are able to localize sounds wherever the sound originates. They also begin to make musical sounds. They are able to sit alone and respond to such simple commands as 'come up' to his mother's outstretched arms. More vocal variety is used in babbling as they add *d, t, ng,* and *w* sounds to it, along with such vowel sounds as *ah* and *eh*. The vocalization of *m-m-m* sounds while crying also begins.

As time progresses, imitation becomes a regular feature of communicative behavior. Children repeatedly imitate their own vocal play. They also imitate adults who use the same sounds they use in their own vocal play. Babbling is now more complex and related to the gratification of needs. Children cease activity when they are spoken to or when they are ordered to discontinue a behavior. They are not particularly interested in environmental sounds outside their immediate surroundings. They have intense interest in words, however. They are most likely using their first two words by now and babble incessantly when alone as they experiment with sound. They produce many sounds simply for the fun of it and frequently repeat words or actions to which adults respond with approval or laughter.

Children at this stage correctly imitate a number of syllables heard in adult vocal stimulation. They figure out several sound groupings and begin producing single words such as "mama" and "dada," since word patterns now become associated with meaning and represent concepts. This process begins the *interiorization of symbols* fundamental to the growth of verbal language.

Very early in their vocalization, children enjoy the sound of their mother's voice and try to imitate what she is saying. This is a very important stage of development that parents should encourage as it provides the basis for an excellent exchange of vocalization activity between adult and child. The child listens and imitates simple sounds as the parents respond to his or her vocalization. This form of interactive behavior stimulates the acquisition of expressive and receptive language, which is indispensable to the normal growth and development of speech and language.

Warning signs

The following are the important warning signs at this stage of development:

- The child does not jabber in response to human voice.
- The child does not use imitation regularly as part of vocal play.
- The child does not show understanding of words made important to him or her through experience (such as the names of food, pets, toys, and family members).
- The child does not obey simple commands.
- The child is not using a few single words (such as "mom," "dad," "dog," and "no").
- The child cannot identify parts of his or her body when prompted.
- The child does not babble and experiment with sounds.
- The child does not progress from babbling to playing with double-syllable sounds.
- The child is unresponsive to the mother's voice and never attempts to imitate what adults are saying.

Twelve Months to Year Two

During this critical period of communicative development, children's speech is structured on what they hear. Toward the end of the second year, children begin an intense use of language to explore their relations with people and things around them. At this stage, they understand fairly specific statements and continue to respond to simple commands and questions, such as 'Give that to Mommy,' or 'Show me a dog,' 'Put your finger on your nose,' or 'Where is your ear?' They also begin, for the most part, to imitate and eventually to generate two-to-four-word sentences. Their longer sentences are usually related to gratification of immediate needs. Their vocabulary is now in the range of two hundred to three hundred words.

The use of complete sentences should be encouraged at this state. The mother should fill in function words when the child is most receptive. She should use narrative or parallel talking; that is, if she understands what the child is saying, she should repeat it using a complete sentence. For example, as the child plays with the piano, mother can say, 'Katie is playing the piano. Very good!' When the child wants something badly, the mother can fill in using more words to explain such as, for example, 'Jane needs some milk now.' This sort of activity provides a good model for the child and helps organize thinking, expressive language, structured sentences, and vocabulary. When the child talks, the caregivers should refrain from responding until the child is finished. The mother should participate in *self-talk*, that is, describe what she is doing at the time, for example, 'Mom is now making the bed,' or 'Andrew is now playing with his truck.'

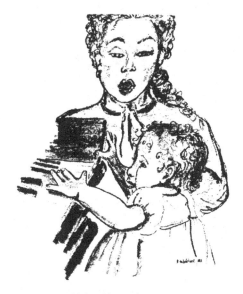

Narrative or parallel talking by mother is important.

Studies have been shown that parents or primary caregivers who engage their children in intensive prelinguistic interaction actually starting at birth help them demonstrate a significant increase in the frequency and quality of their vocalization abilities. (Barnes et al., 1983; Walsh and Greenough, 1976). These children also continue throughout their development to display greater and more lasting gains in communication than those who have been deprived and neglected.

Warning signs

If parents or caregivers do not observe the above-mentioned behaviors and find that their child cannot follow simple and oral directions without visual cues, cannot repeat phrases, or has a vocabulary of less than two hundred words at this stage of development, they should be concerned and seek professional help at the earliest opportunity.

Year Three

Children are now able to follow more complicated instructions and are developing an understanding of complex meanings. There is a marked increase in the use of nouns, which are employed more frequently than verbs, which is then followed by the addition of more adjectives and finally by adverbs as vocabulary exceeds three hundred words. Indeed, most of the phonemes necessary for vocal communication have been acquired by now.

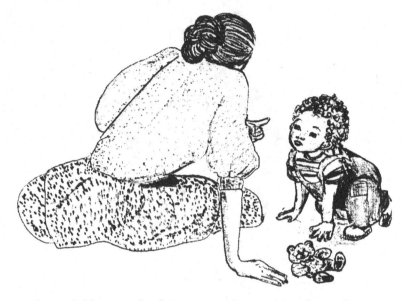

By age three, children are developing an understanding of complex meanings.

Children are fascinated with the use of language and listen carefully to it. They refer to themselves by name. They have become independent and may refuse to be distracted by sounds that are of no interest to them. In other words, they begin to listen selectively, responding to those sounds that are of immediate interest while ignoring those they consider unimportant. In addition, they are now familiar with tense (ex., "sing" as opposed to "sang."; "give" as opposed to "gave") and the appropriate use of the singular and plural forms of words.

Warning signs

Problems may be present if the child:

- Cannot locate the source of sound in the immediate environment
- Cannot understand and use each words as "bring", "go", "me", "big" etc.
- Is unable to follow directions
- Is not alerted by mother's footsteps before seeing her
- Has his or her expressive ability noticeably restricted.

Year Four

Children continue to increasingly exhibit a working knowledge of the rules that govern language. They have a speaking vocabulary of approximately 1, 500 words and a comprehension level which exceeds 5,600 words. Their sentence structure now resembles that of an adult, averaging 5.2 words in length. They are talkative and become truly social beings, with the ability to express emotions verbally. They become aware that phoneme sequences make up meaningful words and that the rules of grammar and syntax determine word order. They are capable of answering questions such as, "What flies?" "What swims?". They use sentences beginning with the word *"how"*.

Warning signs

Problems may be present if the child:

- is unable to give a connected account of experiences
- is unable to carry out two simple directions at a time
- is not talkative
- is not sociable or is withdrawn
- is insensitive to sound
- falls noticeably behind in the development model mentioned so far

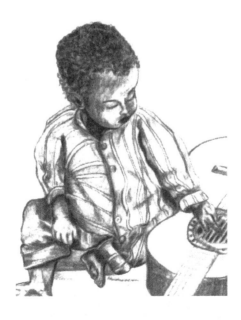

Year Five

By the time children reach five years of age, they adequately express their needs, and their sentences are longer. They have now developed an understanding of the rules that govern language, and the foundation has been properly laid for the intricate variations of adult language. Children can use grammatically correct sentences, which now contain an average of five to seven words. They are conversant with a vocabulary of about two thousand two hundred words, but their comprehension far exceeds this expressive vocabulary. They are starting to develop concepts, especially *that which involves numbers.*

In addition, by this age, children have developed the art of asking questions to get clarification. They constantly ask, 'What is this?' 'Why is that?' 'Why? Why? Why . . . ?' and, most importantly, 'Why not?' They are able to tell a short story and express their feelings and emotions. They identify the time of day and are beginning to understand the concepts of safe versus unsafe. They describe objects by their function. They ask for the specific meaning of words and are able to correct their own errors when learning to pronounce new words. With normal speech development, children at this age can adequately express their needs and use increasingly longer sentences.

Warning signs

Problems may be present if the child

- cannot carry on a simple conversation
- has speech that is stilted, unimaginative, very hard to understand, or generally monotonous (which indicates that the communication system has not developed with the spontaneity of the normal child's communicative skills)
- has no language structure from which to draw so that every new word is a lesson in itself that has to be taught. This usually results in the child being two to four years behind in reading and writing ability by the time he or she reaches junior high school.

School Age

At this stage of development, children show an interest in reading. It is not until hearing children learn to read that a visual symbol system begins to influence further language development and its elaborations (Frisina, 1959). Children are now able to read at the rate of approximately four hundred words per minute, and they speak at a rate of about one hundred and thirty words per minute. Characteristic patterns of speech have been established.

The intricate variations of adult language become evident at this stage as children are now equipped to speak the language of their home, school, and community. They have fine-tuned speech to the point that they can adequately reproduce what they hear. They also begin to show signs of handedness when using crayons or pencils but are not quite certain yet about the concept of "left" and "right."

Articulation is also very important at this stage. Children realize that they must reproduce words they hear with accuracy if they are to be understood. Proper articulation is achieved through listening carefully to the spoken word. However, if listening skills are poorly developed, there may be many errors in sound production as the child is unable to make the correct associations between letter representations and the spoken word. Further, improper articulation may influence reading skills as well. A study by Weaver et al. (1960), using the *Gates Reading Readiness Test* and articulation tests as measures of performance, confirmed a positive relationship between reading readiness and competency in speech, although a causal factor was not determined.

Through the process of effective and productive listening, children have refined an aural—oral language system before he enters the classroom for formal instruction. However, it is important that as they get older, they are exposed to more language stimulation so that neural circuits are pruned into a left hemisphere pattern of specialization for language.

Under normal developmental conditions, by the time children enter school, they have absorbed the language model of their culture and can successfully negotiate their way around that elaborate system of abstract symbolic coding called language for the expression of ideas and concepts that satisfy their escalating needs. They are certainly capable of following complicated commands. Their speech is adequately developed so that there is a noticeable lengthening of sentence structure, and they speak with grammatical correctness if they have been provided with an appropriate model.

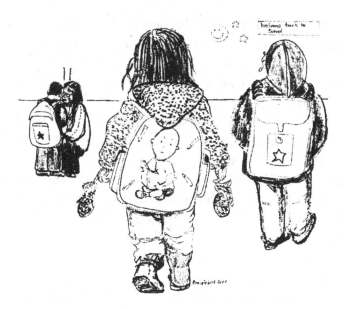

By now, the child has absorbed the language model of the culture.

Language is closely related to children's ability to think abstractly. Burns (1999) observed that for many children, the ability to acquire those building blocks of language is natural and effortless, and all four areas (phonology, semantics, syntax, and pragmatics) combine to make the child a successful communicator on entering school. *For children who have acquired language effortlessly, their solid foundation of oral language prepares them well for their next challenge— learning to read.*

Warning signs

Children with defective hearing or listening skills, may often be characterized as slow, inattentive, and antisocial by refusing to participate in group activities in school. They may often be referred to as dull or even mentally *challenged* while they conceal the extent of their hearing deficiency. In the classroom, the teacher needs to be on the alert for children who are prone to frequent inattentiveness, lack of concentration, below par academic performance, frequent colds, and earaches. Although symptoms of hearing loss may be illusive and may vary with age, parents and teachers must be aware of the warning signs that point to communication difficulties.

Parents are advised to seek professional guidance at the very first sign of abnormal communicative behavior. Whatever the indicator if your child has even one of the warning signs mentioned in the above paragraph, a visit to the physician or hearing clinic is the best investment that can be made in the child's communication development, especially since some children may exhibit what may be regarded as normal auditory functioning and yet still have concealed hearing impairment.

Summary

The development of language perception proceeds in stages. In the early years, environmental sounds form an integral part of the child's waking environment. Children must be shown how to listen selectively and appreciate the sounds around them. The ability to listen effectively is directly related to his ability to acquire speech and language skills appropriately. Children eventually learn what sounds have meaning and how they are used symbolically to communicate ideas and to formulate those ideas into words.

Caregivers particularly must laugh, talk, and read to their children as well as encourage them to communicate at every opportunity possible. Children must be included in such activities as listening to music and the sounds of nature. They need to be constantly exposed to meaningful, pleasant stimuli, which in turn stimulate learning. By watching, hearing, touching, and feeling, children learn about the things around them. All of these activities are important, not only to the normal development of effective listening skills but to the development of speech, language, and a sound intellect.

*Adapted from Daniel R. Boon, *Speech and Language Development in Normal Children*, University of Denver.
Adapted from "The Utilization of Supportive Personnel in Speech Correction in the Public Schools," Phase Two, Rural Communities (J. Alpiner, University of Denver, Project Director).

Chapter 3

What to Do About a
Child's Hearing Impairment

Opinions as to what recourse should be taken when parents discover that their child has a hearing problem vary widely. Many concerns overwhelm caregivers as they try to come to terms with the initial shock of the child's hearing disability. They often ask themselves questions such as these: Will he ever learn to talk? Is she really hearing impaired or is it a mistake with the equipment? Does this mean it is like he is retarded? What will people say? Will she have to wear a hearing aid for the rest of her life? Will all of those loud sounds hurt her ears and make her hearing worse? Will other kids tease him?

The best advice in such circumstances is to seek professional guidance from the most suitable sources available at the earliest opportunity. This applies at any age since today even newborns can be assessed and assisted. The rational is that the earlier the hearing loss is recognized and treated, the better the chances that the treatment will be effective and that the problem will be less severe for the child. The time of onset of hearing loss, the degree of hearing difficulty, and the psychological factors connected with the disability all have important bearing on the speech development of the child (Garrison and Force, 1965). The longer a problem remains undetected and untreated, the harder it will be for the child to develop normal communication skills.

Who are the professionals most likely to provide the necessary direction to caregivers under these circumstances? They are the following:

- family doctor or pediatrician
- audiologist
- otologist
- educator
- caregiver

Of course, caregivers themselves have a key role to play in the process.

Family Doctor or Pediatrician

As mentioned in chapter 2, if as a caregiver you suspect your child has even one warning sign of a hearing problem, arrange for him or her to have a complete physical examination, including a thorough ear, nose, and throat examination by the family physician or a pediatrician. Hearing may be impaired by so many unsuspected physical ailments and not necessarily directly related to the auditory system. Approximately 20 percent of children with hearing problems from birth also have problems with eyes, the nervous system, and the heart (Bete, 1978). Therefore, it is important for the physician to examine the child thoroughly for possible related problems as well. The physician may then refer the child for further examination to an otologist or audiologist if there are suspicions of auditory involvement.

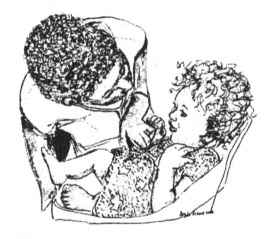

A complete medical examination is necessary, including ears, nose, and throat.

Otologist

An otologist (otolaryngologist) is an MD who specializes in the diagnosis and medical treatment of ear, nose, and throat diseases. As a specialist, an otologist may be able to state the cause of the hearing loss after assessment, at which point he or she may recommend surgery, drugs, or further specialized investigation. Some or all of the child's hearing may be restored by medical or surgical means, depending on what is causing the disorder. Medication is generally used to treat infections of the middle and outer ear. Surgical procedures are at times useful in correcting such conditions as follows:

- structural malformation of the ear
- perforated eardrums

- destroyed bones in the middle ear
- infections

It is the duty of the otologist to provide follow-up care until he or she is satisfied that no further middle ear disease or hearing loss is likely to occur. If inner ear nerve deafness is the problem, the child is systematically evaluated for subtle changes in auditory behavior and for stability in hearing sensitivity. Hearing losses from birth generally do not respond to medication. In order to have correct measurements of hearing levels, the child should visit an audiologist.

Audiologist

When a child has hearing problems of any kind the role of the audiologist is a vital one. The audiologist contributes information on the degree and nature of the hearing loss, the auditory behavior of the child, and the development of the child's hearing status. He or she is specially trained to evaluate and (re)habilitate individuals with hearing problems. In order to determine the extent and nature of the hearing problem the child has, the audiologist performs a test known as an *audiogram* (which checks pure tone and speech levels of hearing) and also measures middle ear function for the existence of middle ear disease.

Figure 3.1.
Audiogram: graphically plots hearing threshold
sensitivity in decibels at each frequency

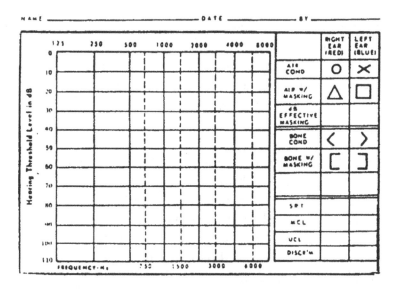

When a hearing loss is significant enough and when medical or surgical procedures are not an option, the audiologist explains the significance of the audiogram in terms of acoustics of speech and speech perception and the factors affecting a specific placement for the child. Upon examination, he or she may recommend a hearing aid. Even infants may be prescribed hearing aids, before the hearing loss affects speech and language development, leading to learning and social maladjustment. Along with the hearing aid evaluation, the audiologist often provide guidance to the caregiver in the planning and maintenance of home programs for development of speech and language skills as well as locating appropriate educational settings for the child.

Early identification and treatment of hearing loss is essential for the development of adequate auditory, linguistic, and social stimulation for speech and language learning, as well as the emotional development of the child. The earlier the intervention occurs, the less defective the child's communication skills will be as he learns to associate sounds with words and words with sentences. The audiologist's assistance is indispensable, therefore, in identifying, coordinating, and utilizing all community resources available for assisting in meeting the specific auditory needs of child.

Educator

Depending on the degree of hearing loss, the child may or may not be able to attend regular classes. If the hearing loss is slight, the child may attend regular classes assisted by such support services as speech and hearing therapy and by individual tutoring, if necessary, by a special teacher. On the other hand, if the hearing loss precludes adequate communication, in the regular classroom setting, even with amplification the child will not be able to attend regular classes.

To prevent the child from falling behind academically and enduring the stigma of social isolation and rejection, it may be necessary to have him or her enrolled in a special day school, private school, special classes, or individual tutoring until communication skills are improved sufficiently for the child to function in a regular classroom setting.

Caregiver

Caregivers are encouraged to be alert to the warning signs related to the child's hearing. If you are a caregiver, familiarize yourself with these warning signs as much as possible. Learn all you can about hearing loss, including its mental, emotional, and social impact on the child's development. Consult your family physician promptly when symptoms appear. Get treatment as quickly as possible to minimize the effects of long-term consequences. Remember that the earlier hearing loss is diagnosed and treated the better the chances that the treatment will be effective and that the problem will be less severe.

If the child is to normally process information, the possibility of hearing loss must be investigated early, especially if the child has had a history of middle ear infection. Remember also that conditions such as allergies can be devastating. With allergies, the child's hearing may be quite normal one day and on other days, it may be inconsistent. There are many factors influencing how a child hears from one day to the next. The season, certain foods, and environmental allergies could all affect the child's hearing and as a result play a crucial role in the way he or she processes information from day to day.

The child may exhibit unresponsive behavior in the classroom as a result of delay in transmission of sound stimuli to the brain caused by one of the above conditions or a temporary hearing loss following an ear, nose, or throat infection. A defective hearing mechanism will affect the child's ability to process information accurately and efficiently. A temporary or permanent conductive hearing loss, for example, can interfere with the acquisition of good perceptual skills which are so vital to the child's intellectual functioning in the classroom. Many studies establish a relationship between chronic otitis media with effusion, learning, and language deficiencies, which influence perceptual and academic achievement (Haggard and Hughes, 1991; Pillsbury et al., 1991).

Teachers often have difficulty understanding why a child suddenly becomes unresponsive and lethargic during instruction. The reason may simply be that he has an ear infection or some similar hearing condition at the time causing internal noise build-up and, hence, delayed transmission of information to the brain. Rather than exploring this possibility, some teachers hastily jump to the conclusion that the child is being uncooperative and has lost interest in studying. They may attribute the child's behavior to laziness, inattentiveness, or to reasons totally unrelated to the real issue.

Authorities often fail to recognize that laziness, inattentiveness, and lack of interest are symptoms rather than the cause of academic failure and frustration. In reality, the child may be experiencing a genuine hearing disorder, which is causing him or her to function with severe limitations. Even a mild, temporary hearing loss resulting from ear infection can reduce the child's ability to process information properly within a noisy classroom environment.

PART

Beyond the Ear

Chapter 4

The Role of the Ear in Processing

We hear sound with our ears. But we must move beyond the ear (*receptive phase of hearing*) to the brain, where meaning is attributed to what we hear (*the perceptive phase of hearing*). The ear is unarguably one of the most intricately designed organs of the human body, and the interrelationship between the ear and the brain is not only one of the most fascinating but also one of the most complex and highly refined processes of the sensory systems.

The ear is involved in our sense of balance and spatial orientation, but its primary function is that of hearing—of taking part in the processing of acoustical information known as speech. The minute details that contribute to the efficiency of this process are intriguing, though not thoroughly understood.

Many questions as to how the ear actually works still baffles the minds of hearing scientists. For instance, how is an incoming experience arriving as complex trains of digitized information, translate into a trace which becomes memory? How does the auditory system process, then store, such vast quantities of information for future recall? How does it organize impulses into meaningful patterns for memory, and how is it retrieved? And how is it capable of ignoring the same bits of information when they are not required, and then immediately retrieve them when required to do so? Furthermore, what actually occurs at the cortical level to order those central auditory abilities into such a latticework of interrelationships we call processing so that incoming impulses could take on meaning? These and scores of other questions are stimulating and are a source of ongoing research and debate.

The ear is more sensitive than the most accurate barometer (instrument that measures changes in atmospheric pressure). It is remarkably suited to respond to changes in air pressure of less than a thousandth of the minimum pressure the most sensitive barometer will record, provided these changes occur rapidly enough. Such changes do in the case of sound so that very small variations in air pressure allow transmission to the ear. These minute surrounding pressure changes are what we know as sound.

The ear's range of sensitivity to sound is incredible. The ear has a dynamic range of about 140dB, that is, its range extends from the weakest signal threshold (ex., the gentle rustle of a leaf by the wind) to a level sufficiently loud to cause pain (ex., an explosion). In other words, it can respond to sound pressures so minuscule as to cause the eardrum to vibrate only about a hydrogen molecule in diameter and transmit that minute sensation to the brain for interpretation. On the other hand, it is capable of withstanding the intense sound pressures of a violent explosion that may register enormous energy outputs.

The ear also responds to a wide frequency (pitch) range as well. Its frequency range is somewhere between 20-20,000 cycles per second (cps or Hz) in the very young child. In the low frequencies, it barely misses detection of the low-frequency rumble of the blood rushing through the veins and arteries of the body or the low-frequency resounding of muscular contractions. On the other hand, we can detect high-frequency signals as high as 20,000 Hz. Sound waves much higher are inaudible to man. Lower animals such as bats do rely on ultrasonic sound to capture their prey. However, it must be said that in humans many of these high frequencies are lost by the onslaught of advancing age.

Hearing as a Constant Activity

Although hearing is such an important sense, it is the one most often taken for granted and neglected. It is only when an individual's hearing ceases to function normally that its worth is truly appreciated. Suddenly, the hearing-impaired individual realizes that he or she now misses a great deal of what is happening around him and begins to feel isolated. The main reason hearing is so often taken for granted is that, unlike vision, we cannot turn it on and off at will to really experience what a genuine hearing loss is like. As a result, we have difficulty truly empathizing with hearing-impaired individuals and understanding the tremendous impact that a hearing loss imposes on them.

Under normal conditions, our ears are never turned off for a moment, even when there is no speech or meaningful acoustic stimuli to process. Our ears constantly respond to the stimulation of sound in the surroundings either at the conscious or subconscious levels. Sound is an integral part of our psychological environment and we are very accustomed to its constant presence. So much so that when individuals are placed in a silent, noise-free acoustic environment such as in dead space, where virtually no sound is perceived except the sounds of one's own body functions, they find that environment discomforting and most difficult to tolerate.

The Role of Hearing in Humans

In many animals, hearing serves a slightly more limited and less sophisticated, albeit equally important function than in humans. For animals, hearing is primarily a reflex-protective activity, where limbs and neck muscles contract and heart rate either increases or decreases in response to sound. Animals depend totally on their built-in alarm system for their survival in the wild. They can readily localize sounds related to danger and take necessary precautions to protect themselves. These stimuli-evoked responses are reflexive responses mediated at the subcortical level of the brainstem and do not require the refined processes at the cortical level, which are more efficiently used and more developed by humans for attributing meaning to sound.

Human hearing on the other hand goes far beyond rudimentary reflexive response of lower animals. Humans recognize, interpret, and attribute meaning to sound thanks to the complex neural functioning of the auditory system, which is capable of processing vast amounts of complex information. Sound in itself is meaningless until meaning is attributed to it by the brain. We assign meaning to the sonic patterns we hear every moment of the day based on objects and events that are meaningful and significant to our human experience.

The ear, therefore, provides the basis for a very complex ordering of skills that end at the brain level, where auditory processing must take place if meaning is to be attributed to sound. Hearing is the first level of perception and constitutes the receptive aspect of sound. Listening transpires beyond the ear, however, and can be regarded as a continuum that ranges from a simple reflex reaction to the ability to process vast amounts of complex information.

Listening is the perceptive use of hearing—a cognitive activity that involves the central auditory nervous system. It is the interpretation of auditory stimulation in a meaningful and discriminative manner by the brain. It bridges the gap between the sounds we hear and that of attributing meaning to those sounds. Neurons are indispensable to this process. As incoming signals are transferred from cell to cell and within cells, they are transformed and modified because billions of neurons build connecting liens for sending messages at great speeds, talking to each other by way of electrical and chemical transmission of signals.

Figure 4.1.

The neuron: a schematic of a neuron showing cell body and processes

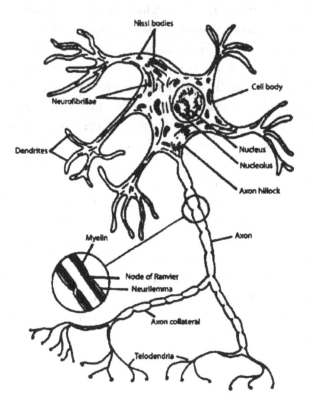

Each neuron is a factory producing specific kinds of chemicals. These chemical signals determine the way we learn and store information for future recall. The central auditory nervous system (CANS) accomplishes elaborate functioning in milliseconds, allowing intricate processes of learning to take place. This processing of complex information is necessary for productive living and provides the basis for dynamic and interactive communication between human beings, without which human survival on this planet would be seriously threatened. *Audition,* therefore, is a basic avenue through which the individual constantly maintains contact with his environment. It is the primary channel for language acquisition and interpersonal relationships.

From Ear to the Brain

Before sound energy reaches the brain, the ear must first transform the acoustic sound wave entering it into an appropriate medium so that it can reach the brain and be understood. The sequence of events by which this is accomplished begins with an acoustic stimulus from the environment. This stimulus must be transformed into an acceptable form of energy that is readable by the central auditory nervous system. This form of energy is the *neural impulse.*

The neural impulses arriving at the brain contain the neural language code of the brain just as a computer programming language is a set of coded instructions that when executed allows the computer to complete a specific task. In the case of neural impulses, the process of transmission is electrochemical in nature. The acoustical environmental energy is transduced into an electrical signal. The electrical signal then becomes a chemical signal when it activates neurotransmission.

Every part of the ear contributes to the efficient transmission of sound to the brain. In fact, the entire auditory system appears to be continuously refining auditory information from the time a signal enters the ear until it reaches the brain for processing. For instance, the primary function of the outer and middle ear is amplification—to make the sound wave intense enough to reach the inner ear successfully. The function of the inner ear is to analyze the signal entering it and then transform this energy into neural impulses for the brain to interpret. Thus the inner ear, having received the acoustic vibrations or sound waves, converts them into neural impulses for transmission to the brain. It does this by the action of the sensory receptors of the cochlea.

Figure 4.2.

Auditory pathway: Diagrammatic illustration of pathway for auditory
impulses from primary centers to the cerebral cortex, showing interconnected
pathways at various levels.

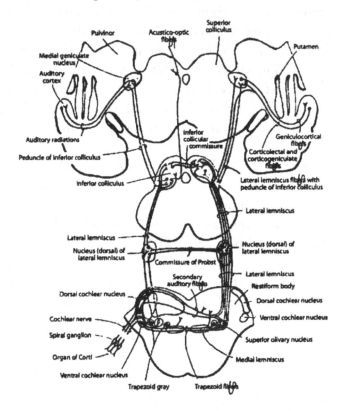

After the sensory receptors of the cochlea convert the waveform into neural impulses, a suitable medium is thus created for transmission of the signal along the auditory nerve to the brain for interpretation. The complexity of the pathway they take to the brain allows for detailed and intricate processing of incoming auditory information. Precise binaural interaction between left and right hemispheres takes place as the signal is transmitted. Various nuclear centers throughout the system receive and integrate signals from the two ears by way of numerous direct and collateral pathways.

This pattern of transmission permits some degree of unrefined signal processing to take place along the way at these junctions en route to the cerebral cortex for final processing. The interconnected pathways at various levels also allow for duplication in diverse parts of the system. This duplication is referred to as *internal redundancy* and is absolutely necessary for the integrity of the entire auditory system since it makes the mechanism highly resistant to total collapse.

The central auditory processes involved must not be regarded as separate entities working independently of each other to accomplish the task of ascribing meaning to the sound; in contrast, they form complex interrelationships. This is what auditory processing or auditory perception is all about. How efficiently the central auditory nervous system ascribes meaning to the auditory stimuli it receives and how speedily it attributes meaning to the constant flow of incoming stimuli, determines how efficiently the whole system works.

The brain is connected directly with every part of the body and is constantly receiving input through the nerves and spinal cord pathways by way of specialized organs of sensation through which it keeps in direct contact at all times with its surroundings. These organs of sensation are the following:

- *the ear*—transmitting noise and sound
- *the eye*—transmitting visual images
- *the nose*—transmitting different odors
- *the tongue*—transmitting different tastes
- *the semicircular canals* in the ear—sending information about position and posture in space
- *the skin*—which consists tiny nerves that tell about touch

The endless stream of information entering the brain every waking moment is mediated in such an organized and efficient manner that the individual is completely aware of his or her surroundings at every consciousness moment.

The auditory system, for example, constantly receives or rejects auditory stimuli at the cortical level. Like the computer, it can receive, sort, store, and retrieve massive amounts of data when called upon to do so. But unlike the computer, it is vastly more sophisticated in its operation. The brain is a complex storage and retrieval system capable of highly discriminatory function. It accepts or rejects what it deems useful or not useful.

Effective listening is the process by which meaning is extracted from auditory stimuli entering the ear that the brain deems appropriate for its use. Once those stimuli are considered relevant, meaning is attributed to them, and we subsequently store, encode, and express our formulated ideas into words based on what the brain has processed.

These complex interrelationships are made possible because billions of interconnected neurons form an integrated central nervous system circuitry exclusively available for processing. For instance, forty billion nerve cells alone are lined up in the hippocampus for storing information from other senses as memory. They are activated as soon as stimuli reach this central processor for interpretation. Once sound stimuli is received by the auditory system, perception takes over and interprets it, organizes it, and sorts it out into meaningful patterns of information for future use. If information is rejected during processing, it is lost as irrelevant and is irretrievable. It is through these fine central auditory nervous system processes that the child makes sense of what he hears and is able to sort, store, and retrieve events from memory as the occasion warrants. This is what is regarded as good perceptual functioning.

When a child listens to the teacher in the classroom, he or she is not in a passive state of mental activity at all but is involved in a profoundly dynamic and energetic undertaking that requires the highest active capabilities of the mind to constantly attribute meaning to what the teacher is saying. This is the function of *inner language* that which gives substance and significance to the input from the ear to the brain. Any disruption of this delicate process can seriously affect the child's ability to ascribe meaning to what he or she hears, resulting in words carrying no symbolic significance. Inner language activity is totally dependent on receptive processes working normally and efficiently. The child's verbal memory and other mental attributes must also be intact if he is to constantly maintain intellectual functioning.

The Efferent Fibers

It is important to note that while there are sensory fibers carrying information to the brain for processing (afferent fibers), there are other fibers carrying information simultaneously away from the brainstem to the cochlea (end organ of hearing) in the inner ear—the (efferent fibers). These ongoing fibers have important implications for hearing and learning—it is believed that they constitute an important feedback loop between the brain and the cochlea.

Figure 4.3.

Olivocochlear bundle—schematized olivocochlear bundle
with efferent and afferent pathways.

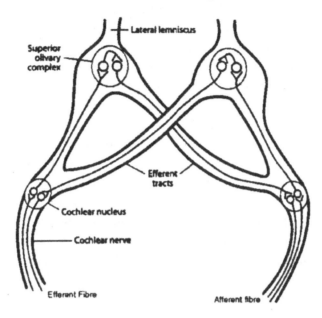

Although this bundle of fibers, called the *olivocochlear bundle,* is relatively small and has limited information-handling capacity, it serves an important function. These fibers decrease neural excitability, making it possible for the ear to make refined and selective judgments as to what information it admits for processing and what information it rejects. The command center overseeing the function of these fibers in the brainstem is called the *reticular activating system* (RAS). It is located in the central part of the brainstem and increases or decreases excitability of most sensory neurons.

The RAS is considered the *alert system* of the brainstem; it helps to keep us on guard and it alerts the cortex, particularly the auditory cortex, to be prepared to process incoming information. The RAS is both selective and discriminatory in its function as it helps the cortex in selecting signals that are of importance while eliminating those that are regarded irrelevant for processing at any given time (Ayres, 1972). It contributes to our ability to memorize, to recall information, to problem solve, to play strategy, and to organize and integrate information once it has been accepted as relevant. Its projections extend upward from the brainstem to the surface of the cerebral cortex.

The RAS receives sensory input from every modality and plays an important role in neural integration. The efficiency with which this system works makes it possible to code and classify not only on the basis of whether the information is auditory or visual, for example, but also on the basis of whether the information is meaningful or meaningless. The RAS facilitates or inhibits sensory transmission at all levels within specific afferent pathways. The process of central auditory processing probably involves an interplay of this system with other systems, such as the *limbic* and *reticular systems (subcortical structures of the brain concerned with emotion and motivation)* as well as the *cerebral auditory cortex*. All of these systems are involved in the process of listening and assigning meaning to incoming information.

Children with learning disabilities display a high degree of distractibility probably due to a deficiency in the function of the RAS. These children seem to operate with a system that is deficient in both its discriminatory and selective functioning. Therefore, the system does not effectively suppress neural excitability as it should; instead, it allows too many sensory signals to be admitted at once to the brain, thus short-circuiting the system with irrelevant information. In other words, it accepts too much irrelevant information for processing, while at the same time processing too little of what may be considered relevant. This condition contributes to the high level of distractibility displayed by the child in the classroom. *They pay fleeting attention to all objects and events impinging on their environment irrespective of relevance.*

If the RAS is not working efficiently because the child's central auditory nervous system is underdeveloped, not having achieved full auditory maturation, this will limit the child's ability to listen selectively. Teachers in the language arts stress the fact that unless children listen effectively, they will develop inadequate verbal sequential memory (the ability to remember sounds and words in their sequential order) and will suffer severely in the production of their oral language skills (Allen, 1969).

Finally, as was already discussed, effective listening involves both the *receptive* and *perceptive* aspects of hearing for good oral production. Auditory speech perception and production are intricately interrelated activities. The listener hears, then he perceives (understands), and finally expresses his perception of what he is thinking in the form of speech. This process can be regarded as the productive aspect of listening. The speaker determines the message content, word order, grammatical structures, rate, intonation, and gestures necessary to make himself meaningfully understood through speech.

If effective communication is to take place, therefore, it is essential that there is adequate reception, perception (interpretation), and production of sound. In the classroom when a child is unable to attribute meaning to what he hears, this dynamic interaction process between what is heard, interpreted, and what is correctly verbalized is disrupted. The persistent result of this is a disruption in the normal development of inner language function in the child—that which gives substance and meaning to what he hears and speaks—which is totally dependent on good receptive processes for its development.

Chapter 5

The Child Who Does Not Understand

Effective listening is the process by which information is decoded and encoded by the brain. Decoding is the process of extracting meaning from auditory stimuli. Humans recognize sound because their brain attributes meaning to the sound it receives as long as inner language—the language of the mind—has been developed. We all hear if there is no impairment of the ear, but to listen effectively means that we have acquired an *inner language* that enables us to constantly attribute meaning and substance to what we hear. We then encode the information received and later express our formulated ideas in words.

As mentioned earlier, when children listen in the classroom, they are constantly assigning meaning to what the teacher is saying because they have learned to integrate experiences into symbolic significance through the process of inner language. It is estimated that up to four million primary and secondary school children in the United States alone may be experiencing some form of listening disorders or auditory processing difficulty in school, which affects their ability to understand information presented. That is, they have a deficiency in inner language that prevents them from attributing meaning appropriately to what they hear.

Most of these children are undiagnosed (Greenwald, 1999). Typically, they respond in the classroom by saying "Huh?" or "What?" or "I don't understand" or, "Repeat that" over and over again. They behave as though they were hearing-impaired when in reality they are not. What causes a child to behave in this fashion? What is it that makes it so difficult for him to understand, when other children seem to grasp concepts so effortlessly?

A number of these children have problems with auditory processing (Geschwind, 1967; Penfield and Roberts, 1959; Russell and Espir, 1961), which involves the neurology of inner language (giving substance, meaning, and significance to what they hear and speak—input and output). Under normal listening conditions, the brain is capable of processing information in milliseconds. How intelligently a child functions within his listening and learning environment such as the classroom, depends on the speed and the efficiency with which auditory processes are executed.

The problem is that many children in today's classrooms are failing to perform these functions with speed and efficiency because of a breakdown in certain neurological processes which hinders them from integrating and organizing incoming stimuli into meaningful patterns of information for academic purposes. They are experiencing what can be characterized as a performance deficiency in auditory reception, which restricts their ability to attribute meaning to what is heard or read.

A central auditory processing disorder is a performance deficiency in auditory signal reception with particular influence on the language processing capabilities of children. It disrupts the delicate, finely tuned precision with which the brain communicates with the ear. Something intercepts the information from the ear to the brain. When this delicate balance is disturbed, critical central abilities are affected. When these abilities fail, the child will perform with less than normal efficiency and is said to be experiencing an auditory processing disorder.

To better understand what such children are experiencing, imagine going into a room with foreign speakers who are conversing in a foreign language. Surely, you hear the words, and some of them may even be familiar to you, but you are unable to make sense of what you hear because you do not understand the rules that govern that language. You lack the knowledge of how the sounds are used to fit together to make up the words of the language. The children's behavior is similar. They cannot understand what they hear because they do not have the necessary proficiency with language concepts to facilitate learning. Consequently, they are often mislabeled by teachers and caregivers as unmotivated or even as lacking intelligence. But the truth is that their behavior frequently has nothing to do with intelligence or motivation; instead, it has to do with the frustration they are experiencing because of a defective auditory channel.

These children's primary difficulty is that of learning through the auditory channel; they cannot make maximum use of what they hear. Something goes wrong between what they hear with the ear and the interpretation of that incoming signal by the brain. This results in enormous difficulty in translating sounds into language and associating sounds that are heard with a language concept. They may have good speech discrimination, but yet may suffer significant deficiency in attributing meaning to what they hear, as a result, they process information slowly and inaccurately. They *mishear* things frequently or behave as though they do not hear what was said at all.

It is believed that the brain of these children, as far as sound processing is concerned, is wired differently and that the neural circuits that support language are poorly connected. Consequently, incoming stimuli are not properly rooted to their appropriate designations in the brain for processing. This problem with signal reception prevents the brain from efficiently discriminating, integrating, and organizing sound into meaningful patterns of information. Whether it is an *auditory integrative deficiency* where the underlying problem is that of comprehending the spoken word as displayed by a deficiency in receptive language skills, or an *auditory output organization deficiency* where the child is unable to sort, plan, or organize an appropriate response to information, the results are the same. Poor storage and retrieval capabilities of the brain, displayed in inadequate receptive, expressive, and integrative language skills on the part of the child.

What is worrying is that these children do appear to have normal listening skills. Upon close inspection, however, certain traits distinguish them from the normal listening children. Even though their hearing is normal, they usually experience difficulty with the following tasks at varying levels of difficulty, depending on the extent of the deficiency:

- localizing the source of information
- comprehending the meaning of environmental sounds
- distinguishing and selecting important stimuli from unimportant stimuli
- combining syllables to form words and combining words to make meaningful sentences

In the classroom, all of these deficiencies manifest themselves in the child's expressive and receptive functional behaviors, exacerbated by inattention, imperfect speech, bewildered and perplexed expression, and inconsistent response to language.

Another clearly delineated problem area for these children is their marked inability to function in the presence of noise, meaning anything superfluous, unwanted, random, or disturbing in the environment. The presence of noise has a debilitating effect on their ability to think, receive information, and properly decode it. In any regular classroom, there are times when noise levels are clearly disruptive and handicapping. When this happens, processing closes down for these children. (More will be said on this later on.)

Children with CAPD characteristically have problems with extracting information in the presence of noise. It is for this reason that their behavior is frequently misconstrued by both teachers and caregivers as a lack of interest in achievement, lack of intelligence, or just plain laziness. Some children have learned to handle these problems by shutting out sound and behaving as though they had a hearing impairment. Others cover their ears and show reduced tolerance for noise in the environment. In general, they devise whatever means possible to conceal their lack of understanding. Such a practice, if allowed to persist, can have serious long-term consequences on their ability to learn.

Furthermore, when one examines the medical history of children with CAPD, it is not uncommon to find a history of early middle ear disease such as serous otitis media with effusion, usually accompanied with a family history of learning difficulties on the mother's or father's side of the family. Research acknowledge that an early history of chronic otitis media with effusion (OME) is associated with a high incidence of learning difficulty, language deficiencies, and attention disorders.

Characteristic Behaviors of the Child Who Does Not Understand

Children with comprehension problems both in and out of the classroom, may frequently say,

- "I don't understand."
- "What did I do wrong."
- "I don't remember."

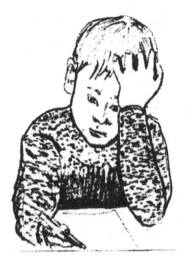

The child may be misunderstood as stubborn or lazy.

When this behavior is exhibited in the classroom, the teacher may say things such as

- "He's lazy."
- "She says she understands, but she doesn't."
- "He never seems to learn or get it right."
- "He should have his hearing tested."
- "I tell him the same thing over and over again, but it doesn't sink in."
- "Her comprehension level seems far below par for her age."
- "I don't know if he is stubborn or if he really doesn't understand."
- "Reading and writing are extremely poor, and he seems to get stuck in the middle somewhere."
- "She has problems with understanding language concepts such as, idioms or homonyms and synonyms.'
- "She has a short memory span."

Hearing in Noisy Conditions

As has been observed earlier, in the classroom, it is not uncommon for noise to reach levels that render learning virtually impossible. When compounded with reverberation caused by poor classroom acoustics, noise is devastating to impaired listeners. It generates distortion, which in turn degrades the quality of spectral speech information, making it difficult to understand the spoken word. Noise inevitably imposes restrictions on the ability to think. Under noisy conditions, children with a central auditory processing disorder may have problems with auditory attention and auditory memory figure-ground extraction. This means that they cannot recall enough of the vital elements of the message because they cannot extract sufficient information from the background noise to make sense of what they hear.

If they cannot make sense of what they hear—which is perception—then what they experience is *imperceptibility*—the inability to structure the mass of information impinging on the auditory system. They are incapable of organizing auditory events so that they can have meaning (Richardson, 1977). As long as noise is present within the learning environment, they will be deficient in predicting and formulating meaning from sentences when information is missing from that message. Many of these children struggle daily in the noisy classrooms in which they function. When such conditions are prevalent, auditory learning is inhibited and all aspects of auditory functioning is impeded, verbal and nonverbal.

But how do normal listening children cope under the same conditions? How do they understand speech when it is spectrally distorted? The threshold of annoyance varies from child to child; some children have higher tolerance levels than others. Generally, since it may not be possible to see the teacher at all times or hear her every word because of the noise levels, normal listening children rely on various avenues that allow them to keep speech in focus despite the noise.

Auditory Closure and Redundancy

One such avenue for comprehension in noise is *auditory closure*. It fills in the missing bits of information that the eye and ear fail to grasp under poor conditions of listening. Auditory closure is the ability to achieve meaning without analysis and to configure as a whole bits of information even though there are gaps in the message received. This is referred to as *redundancy*. The normal listener relies on the redundancy of the message—the abundance of informational cues inherent in the message such that if parts of the message are omitted, that omission would not distort the overall meaning of the message received.

Normal listeners, therefore, do not have to hear every detail of a message to understand it. Auditory closure allows them to rely heavily on the context of the message under the most difficult listening conditions. Normal listeners are also good at making guesses and identifying words that are mumbled or enmeshed in noise to extract meaning. They do this by relying on the brain's ability to exploit harmonic structures of speech and those subtle but distinctive vocal qualities that distinguishes one speaker's voice from that of another. By doing so, they filter information more efficiently and can interpret it more intelligently at the brain level.

Children with auditory processing difficulties either do not have this facility or are incapable of maximizing on auditory closure to their advantage for extracting meaning from degraded speech. Children with CAPD have a remarkably low tolerance for noise. In the regular classroom, where efficiency is demanded of every child, noise can and does affect childrens' ability to process. As a rule of thumb, teachers should be aware that whenever they need to raise their voice above the level of the background noise in order to be understood as little as a meter away from the nearest listener, then acceptable noise levels have been exceeded in that area.

Selective Attention and Problems with Decoding

The noisy classroom environment limits children's capacity for selective attention. Too often, by the time the information reaches the ear, it is too fragmented and degraded by environmental conditions for them to make sense of it. Overwhelmed by too many stimuli, they become incapable of focusing attention on the primary source of information, which is teacher's voice. Because the incoming stimuli are undecipherable, the children, therefore, find it difficult to attach meaning to what they hear so that they cannot make maximum use of it for academic purposes. Extracting meaning from auditory stimuli entering the ear is one of the essential performance criteria children need in order to survive in the classroom. It is a basic survival skill—a skill absolutely necessary for them to succeed.

Because these children are required to expend so much listening time while trying to process correctly, they fatigue easily, and listening eventually becomes a stressful experience. When this happens, learning cannot take place. The alert classroom teacher should always be aware of the point where attention is compromised.

As decibel levels (intensity) rise in the classroom, loudness perception increases even more rapidly than the listener perceives. For example, a sound of ninety decibels (large truck at close range) is ten times stronger than a sound of eighty decibels (normal buzz of city noise). And yet a sound of 110-120 decibels (pneumatic drill at full blast) is hundred times stronger than that some eighty decibels buzz of the city noise. There is an exponential increase in loudness as we reach the higher end of the loudness scale. The implications are as follows: in the classroom, that portion of the speech spectrum on which the child relies for speech intelligibility is unfortunately that portion that is most severely affected by the background noise of the classroom. Most of the frequency bands contributing to the understanding and intelligibility of speech are relatively easy to distort by background noise because of the low level of speech power these bands contain. Any slight increase in classroom noise essentially masks these weak consonant sounds that contribute about 60 percent or more to the intelligibility of the speech we hear.

Figure 6.1 A.
English speech sounds distributed across frequency.

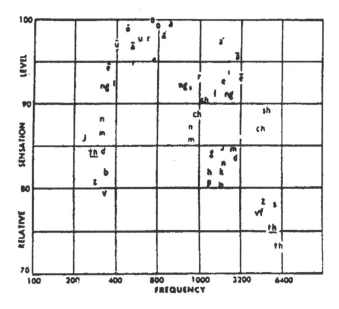

Figure 6.1 B.
Relative intensities of English speech sounds.

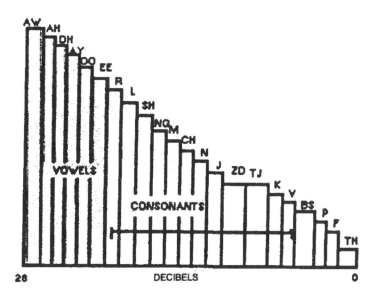

It is primarily the mid-to-high frequency consonant sounds of speech that provide most of the acoustic information necessary for understanding what we hear in speech. Without them, speech becomes muffled and unintelligible. When consonant sounds are masked by noise, it is like trying to make sense of what a person is saying with his or her mouth covered. These distorted codes of information arrive at the child's brain, virtually impossible to decipher, and consequently instructions from the teacher make no sense to the child at all under such conditions. The child is, therefore, forced to ask to have things repeated. Is it any wonder then that he says, "What?" or "Huh," or "I don't understand" repeatedly?

As has been observed earlier, children with decoding problems seem to get too little information altogether in order to make sense of what they are hearing. Their attention-filtering capabilities are greatly diminished in highly competitive listening conditions. In most cases, when these children are removed from the source of noise, there is remarkable recovery in their performance. It must be pointed out, however, that when an auditory decoding deficiency such as this becomes extreme enough, the child may have difficulty processing even under ideal listening conditions.

Aspects of Reading

Problems of auditory decoding imposes limitations in all areas of phonemic awareness and discrimination and restrict the development of normal language and reading abilities. There is generalized inability in the use of oral language, with reading especially affected since hearing is to speech what vision is to reading. Children who have these problems are slow as they read, stumbling on sounds and words as they transduce the visual word into its auditory equivalent. In the process, they tend to lose their place on the page easily.

To compensate, many of them may be seen pointing with their fingers as they struggle along over the page, producing individual sounds and attempting to blend them into words. This is a form of dyslexia, where children have great difficulty with whole-word recognition or learning to read from a global approach. They must break words down into individual sounds and then blend them into words because they find it difficult to retain entire sequences of letters that form whole words as they attempt to read. But they can learn individual sounds to rely on for blending into words. This is time consuming and requires much patience on the part of the teacher.

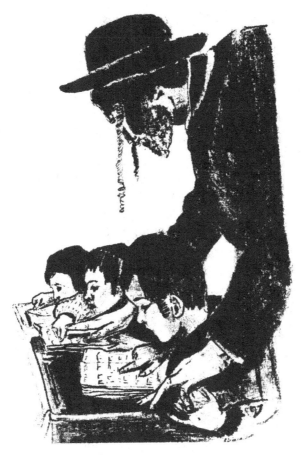

They may be seen pointing to retain their position on the printed page.

Some children use a line guide while reading to maintain their position on the printed page. This is because they tend to move their head rather than their eyes across the page or are frequently seen reading while propping their head on their hands, which indicates fatigue as they struggle to facilitate the blending of auditory and visual components of sounds into words.

In these situations, the child suffers significantly, because, as researchers at Rutgers University have pointed out, in order to read well, the brain has only a few thousandths of a second to translate each visual symbol into its proper sound since reading is a visual symbol superimposed on an auditory language system. Most children can process such sounds in less than forty milliseconds. Language-impaired children, however, may require up to five hundred milliseconds to process the same sounds fast enough to speak fluently or to read properly (Holtz, 1998). Children with auditory decoding problems are in this category. They experience the following difficulties:

- When reading, they are unable to process visual information on the page fast enough to scan letters on that page.
- They frequently experience difficulty separating sounds embedded in speech into distinct units fast enough to comprehend.
- They may be having difficulty "mapping a single letter or cluster of letters to a sound" Holtz (1998).
- Their brains process information too slowly (perceptual speed) to distinguish between sounds from which words are composed.
- Auditorily, they cannot identify and sound out phonemes properly.
- They cannot retain a visual sequence.

I have heard teachers observe that some children in such circumstances just seem to get stuck on a particular sound and struggle to proceed with the rest of the text, but just cannot move ahead.

Most of these children are of normal intelligence with no significant visual problems or visible signs of emotional disturbance that may be contributing to their difficulty in reading. But they cannot read because they cannot store visual or auditory images long enough for immediate recall. As has been observed, reading is primarily a visual symbolic system superimposed on an auditory scheme. If a child cannot integrate these two modalities normally, he or she will suffer disturbance in reading, finding reading a difficult challenge that is to be avoided at all costs.

When all of this is compounded by noise in the environment, one can see how difficult it must be for these children to survive in the regular classroom under conditions of increased competition. As they struggle to keep up with the teacher and their peers, they miss large chunks of the vital information imparted by the teacher, so they simply have difficulty remembering what they have been taught.

This struggle for survival in the classroom often leads authorities to the inaccurate conclusion that the child is lazy or of low intelligence. On intelligence tests that require both nonverbal and verbal scales to obtain an accurate IQ score, this child would invariably score higher on the nonverbal portion than on the verbal measures. But it must be remembered a low score may simply be a reflection of language retardation rather than an index of the overall low mental capacity of the child. Indeed, the child may show superiority in other nonverbal mechanical abilities. In such nonverbal areas, he or she may well be in a better position to compete on equal terms with more verbal peers.

Chapter 6

The Child Who Forgets

You may hear the child say things such as:

- "I forgot."
- "Would you repeat that?"
- "Huh?"
- "What did you want me to do?"
- "I didn't hear the beginning of what you said."

You may hear the teacher or caregiver say about the child:

- "He speaks incorrectly, mixes up specific letter sounds, and misspells words."
- "She does poorly in noise."
- "He often asks to have things repeated and can't seem to remember what he was told even though his hearing has been tested normal."
- "She can't seem to talk right and never pronounces words correctly."
- "She has problems finding the right word to say."
- "He has problems with phonics."
- "She never pays attention."
- "She never seems to complete assignments."
- "Forgets the question when called on in class."
- "He must have a hearing problem."

These are the warning signs of CAPD. Children who forget easily are those to generally get too little information or too much information at once when listening, especially in noise. Thus they forget quickly what little they have heard. This condition is at times referred to as an *auditory memory span* disorder. Auditory memory span refers to the amount of information a child is capable of retaining in proper sequence for the purpose of immediate action or recall. A disorder in this area of processing is caused by forgetting what was said by not understanding it well enough to store it appropriately for future recall.

Often, children with auditory memory deficiencies are considered underachievers or even learning failures, since their performance does not measure up to their intellectual capacity. They are described as forgetful, inattentive, disorganized, and prone to daydream, lacking the focus and concentration necessary to succeed. Teacher becomes frustrated with them because these children quickly forget what they have been told. They cannot recall words easily for verbal or oral expression. It is not uncommon for them to forget questions when called upon by the teacher in the classroom. They simply do not remember what was asked. Memory-based skills such as word recall and retrieval and sequential memory so important to the process of self-expression are significantly affected here.

Because these problems are associated with auditory verbal comprehension, the expressive language of certain children with CAPD tends to be concrete, with deficiencies in both content and syntax. These children generally rely heavily on memory for concrete things, which is, unfortunately, sometimes mistaken for lack of general intelligence. They cannot recognize relationships between experiences, and this affects their ability to generalize or to think abstractly and to form logical conclusions. Whenever the teacher ask them to do a new task, they are usually slow in starting and may wait until others have started in order to mimic what they see without conceptualizing the task. If they do not catch on to the rules of the activity immediately, it is only after repeated trials that they can accomplish the task. At times, they may easily give up altogether, finding the task too difficult. Their inability to predict consequences of behavior may cause them to appear disrespectful or even obstinate as they misread the feelings and attitudes of others. Because of this, they respond inappropriately to events around them. Consequently, they tend to be socially isolated as peers, teachers, and caregivers often regard them as naïve and unintelligent.

In addition, because these children are limited in their interpretation of the intended or implied meaning of what is said, they have difficulty understanding figurative speech. This results in overly literalistic interpretation of ideas and concepts, since their thinking is generally at an elemental level, and they are severely restricted mentally in dealing with the subtleties of language. I once asked a child if he understood the meaning of "The grass is always greener on the other side." He replied, "Which side?" In another instance, a teacher asked a student to interpret what the statement "Those plans are still in the air," meant to her. She replied, "Someone is planning an airplane flight somewhere." Another teacher showed a child a picture of people shopping in a mall and asked him to explain what he thought the people were doing. The child pointed to the picture and replied quite emphatically, "Look, they are right here, here in the picture!" In response to the same picture, other children in the same class readily exclaimed, "Oh, they are shopping in the mall!" and "They are buying this or that."

Certain children with nonverbal learning disorders do not perceive interrelationships in situations and may behave inappropriately in responding to normal everyday events. On the other hand, children with a verbal expressive disorder may grasp meaning but cannot express their ideas in words because of an expressive language deficiency. In both cases, verbal disabilities resulting from central auditory nervous system dysfunction are responsible for their inappropriate behavior.

Interestingly, the child mentioned above is the same child that always raises his hand first in class in response to a question from the teacher. But as the teacher turns to him for a response, the boy invariably stares vaguely at her and says nothing. What is going on here? Why do some children behave in this manner? These children may be suffering from what is known as a *reauditorization disorder*. They have difficulty recalling words and become frustrated in communication because they cannot remember how to say what they have in mind. These children must be taught how to retrieve the words they want to use through proper storage and retrieval methods.

These examples above serve to provide a typical illustration of the overly literalistic interpretation of ideas and a failure by certain children to grasp the complexity and subtlety of language. One reason for some children's inflexibility with language concepts is the difficulty they have linking incoming information with information previously learned, which limits their ability to adequately generalize to new situations. In some of these children, there is no consistent pattern of behavior from one task to the next to suggest any degree of generalizing capability, which is so essential to concept formation. Every task seems to be new and unrelated and has to be learned from scratch.

Children with CAPD may have severe difficulty applying the basic rules of language to sound (ex., associating letters of the alphabet with sounds). They may also have problems with the following:

- grammar and semantic concepts
- relationships among or between words
- antonyms (words with opposite meaning)
- synonyms (different words with same meaning)
- homonyms (words sounding alike with different meaning)

Such restrictions in verbal intelligence limit these children's ability to generalize, make abstract associations, draw rational conclusions, and to compete successfully in those tasks that require abstract and symbolic association. This is due to the close relationship between general language usage and abstract thought. Noticeably lacking is their ability to generalize from one situation to another and to make appropriate association between things. At the same time, conceptualization does not merely refer to the ability to abstract, but it is also associated with the ability for categorical reasoning (Johnson and Myklebust, 1971).

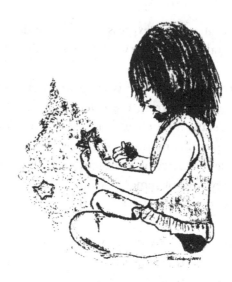

Conceptualization involves categorical reasoning

Children with CAPD who cannot conceptualize, generally experiences a breakdown in categorical reasoning and do not have the capacity to generalize beyond the immediate event. It is thus difficult for them not only to infer beyond the literal event through generalization, but in general to engage in abstract thinking and creative activities altogether—to problem solve, make comparisons, and successfully manipulate language for academic purposes. All of this is because these children have not made the normal progression from perception to abstraction and then on to generalization.

Writing

A child who cannot read, cannot write. When children with CAPD write, their letters are poorly formed and not legible, with inadequate space between them and between words, indicating poor phonic discrimination. Their ability to sequence and arrange sounds that form words in their proper order, as well as synthesize the parts of speech to form a whole sentence, is severely affected (Barr and Carlin, 1972). The explanation is that they may be unable to retain and recall a series of sounds in sequence within words. Severe auditory discrimination problems may also be reflected in their writing if they cannot distinguish fine discrimination differences in consonants such as *b* and *d* and words such as "ear" and "air" and "coal" and "cold," "found" and "fond," "wish" and "which."

These children also have difficulty following commands since they cannot retain a series of simple instructions in sequence. In addition, they have serious problems taking class notes because they cannot remember what they hear while they struggle to write.

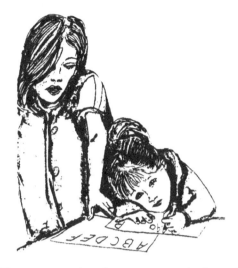

Writing is a task as letters are poorly formed.

Note taking in class is often a serious problem. These children's handwriting skills are generally so poorly developed and illegible that they struggle to transcribe letters on the page while at the same time attempting to keep pace with the teacher and their peers. They are bound to miss large chunks of information that is critical to understanding. This creates confusion, causing the child to respond sporadically to information, particularly when instructions are complex, and thus constantly ask the teacher to repeat what was said. Note taking is difficult, therefore, because they forget information readily. They are too busy trying to keep pace with the teacher to remember what they heard.

They hear normally but do not interpret the sounds accurately because they are easily overwhelmed by too much information at once as they struggle to process the string of rapidly successive sounds that make up speech. Becoming overwhelmed, they fatigue easily from listening and withdraw. Valuable learning time is wasted when these problems go unrecognized.

As was mentioned earlier, children with inner language deficiency—especially those with receptive disturbance, input problems, and problems that center around comprehension, presents a generalized disturbance because of its severity. Much of this disturbance is attributed to the close connection that exists between ordinary language usage and abstract thought. With a defective inner language system, thinking, ideas, and concepts are processed by these children slowly and differently.

These children's basic perception of the world is different, which is reflected in the image they project. As a result, they encounter enormous difficulty just in the simple process of growing up. They are less mature, more protected, less adventurous, and less creative in behavior. They generally appear withdrawn, socially isolated, and deprived, which reflects severe problems with social perception.

Chapter 7

The Child Who Is Disorganized and Confused

I have intentionally combined these two topics—confusion and disorganization—because they share many characteristics. Confused and disorganized children may frequently say:

- "I can't do it. It's too difficult."
- "Explain that to me again."
- "I am confused."
- "Repeat it, I am confused."
- "I get confused when more than one person is talking at once."
- "I can't do more than one thing at once."
- "I can't find my homework."
- "I don't know where I have put my notes."
- "I can't say it right."
- "I don't know what to say."
- "I don't want to play. They make fun of me."
- "She has no friends and her behavior is antisocial."
- "I can't seem to find anything."
- "I can't make sense of what I have written."

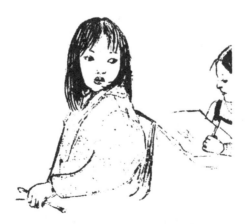

Child waits on others to see how a task is done before proceeding.

Their teachers and caregivers may say the following:

- "This child is slow to respond, waits for others to see how a task is done before attempting it herself."
- "He has problems reading and spelling."
- "She never wants to take part in activities with other kids, especially anything that has to do with music."
- "She can't seem to do more than one thing at a time."
- "He always gets confused when more than one person is talking at once."
- "She fatigues easily when trying to listen or performs poorly after listening for prolonged periods of time."
- "He speaks and writes jumbling words without making appropriate pauses between them."
- "She is messy and disorganized."
- "He has difficulty taking notes and organizing them."
- "He can't follow directions containing several parts."
- "She doesn't seem to say what she means and generally expresses herself poorly."
- "He is clumsy, awkward, and uncoordinated. He is always knocking over things or tripping over everything."
- "He never completes his assignments."
- "She has problems speaking. She makes many grammatical errors in her speech and writing."
- "His spelling and writing are poor even though it appears that he understands what he wants to say."

Organization *Deficit*

The ability to plan, sort, and organize information into a logical sequence requires the participation of the front of the cerebral hemisphere (the forehead area), which is the *prefrontal cortex of the brain*—the seat of 'high executive function,' as it is called. The maturing of this area allows children to exercise choices and control over what they regard as appropriate behavior. It assists the brain in organizing an appropriate response to all incoming stimuli. When this area of the brain has not achieved a proper level of maturity, children's academic performance suffer because they are unable to hold on to incoming information long enough to formulate an appropriate response to it.

Children who behaves in a disorganized manner are said to have an *output-organization deficit*. Their difficulty resides in the neural task of planning, sorting, organizing, and formulating an appropriate response to the information they receive. The problem is reflected most significantly in the encoding phase of linguistic behavior. In other words, their expressive language tends to lag behind their receptive language (understanding) skills. They understand perfectly what they have heard, but they have difficulty retaining, planning, and organizing the stimuli they receive into an appropriate response.

This inadequacy in recalling and expressing information stems from the fact that these children cannot retain a sequence of sounds within words and words within sentences long enough which is essential for retrieval and expression. This inability is bound to affect the proper storage of information by the brain, and, therefore, it influences the brain's ability to scan and retrieve information for an appropriate response. The brain itself is a complex storage and retrieval system that mandates that information be properly stored and organized in order to be retrieved when demanded.

Disorganized children are often handicapped in the regular classroom because of their inability to plan and organize information appropriately. What is more disturbing is that often no evaluation has been done to determine whether this child has the basic tools necessary to succeed in a particular classroom setting and whether the child's placement can truly be considered *selective placement* so that it best accommodates his or her particular auditory needs. When this happens, the child functions at a significant disadvantage in the classroom since no thought has been given to the conditions that best facilitate his or her learning.

These noticeable limitations in auditory memory and retrieval skills are displayed in expressive auditory language function, leading to educational challenges, psychosocial problems, and other forms of social and intellectual maladjustment. The encouraging thing about an *expressive language deficiency* of this nature is that it shows remarkable plasticity in response to proper management as compared to a *receptive language deficiency* (understanding), which is comparatively resistant to change and in which aberrant behaviors are more firmly entrenched.

Expressive language deficiency can be markedly improved through linguistic emersion that includes frequently planned presentations of structured language (to help the child become familiar with correct language structure), coupled with persistent caregiver-child verbal interaction. Such a program must be deficit-specific, tailored to the child's needs, and geared to the mental and language levels of the child. As with all remedial programs, it must contain built-in components to measure progress throughout the learning process. If done right, the results can be remarkable.

Confusion

Similarly, children who appear constantly confused may experience difficulty executing simple tasks independently or simultaneously. This confusion may be attributed to poor interhemispheric transfer of information between the right and left hemispheres of the brain. The neurology of verbal behavior differs from that of nonverbal behavior in that the left hemisphere of the brain is responsible for verbal function and the right for nonverbal function.

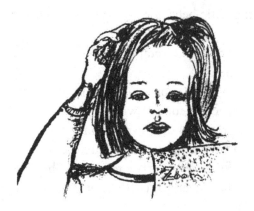

Child appears constantly confused and is unable to execute simple tasks independently.

The problem is that many simple tasks require the simultaneous use of both sides of the brain to carry them out smoothly and efficiently. If information from one side of the brain is disrupted and does not cross efficiently to the other, the child will experience difficulty learning because of a receptive disturbance in the form of auditory confusion—a breakdown in the organization and selective processes of the system, such that the child is incapable of structuring the mass of incoming impulses into a meaningful, coherent pattern for learning.

These auditory input deficiencys are debilitating in nature. They have a tendency to severely modify and reduce children's capacity to manage information efficiently, thus limiting their total learning experience. This problem manifests itself particularly in how these children relate to such concepts as time (seconds, minutes, hours, days, seasons), space—time-relationships, left—right orientation, and quantification measurements (greater than, less than). All of these conceptual areas are markedly affected because of a receptive disturbance. Since receptive disturbances have a tendency to be of generalized severity, they affect not only the children's academic performance, but also often their emotional and psychological adjustment as well, eventually disturbing ego development. Consequently, their relationships are affected, and they never seem to reach full social and intellectual maturity, always lacking the tools for adjustment and understanding.

In the classroom, these children are easily confused when trying to accomplish more than one task simultaneously (*multitasking*). For instance, they may be trying to take dictation from the teacher who is walking around the classroom as she talks—which means they must track her while taking notes—and also simultaneously trying to decipher information from the chalkboard or from what she is saying. Listening can become a frustrating task under these circumstances. It is not uncommon to see some children withdraw from these situations and simply give up or cover their ears to block out sound and isolate themselves.

Unlike children with *auditory decoding* problems, who are receiving too little information to process effectively and, therefore, forget what they hear, these children are receiving too much information (information overload) at once and are unable to selectively focus on information of importance coming from the teacher.

In summary, all of the children with perceptual difficulties described so far display a combination of the following characteristics in varying degrees of severity—maturational lags, difficulties in integration (expressed primarily in reading tasks where visual and auditory integration is necessary), short memory span, difficulties in auditory sequencing, and perceptual speed and general delays in expressive and receptive language skills. These deficiencys are reflected in all aspects of their academic performance and communicative behavior, which significantly contributes to their distractibility in the classroom and seriously influence their ability to learn.

Chapter 8

Noise And The Mind
Lost In The Classroom

Our children come into this world bombarded with noise from every quarter, and at every level, every waking moment of their lives. We live in a society inundated by noise. There is noise everywhere. Our society has paid a high price in its haste toward modernization. In our rapidly growing metropolis, noise pollution continues to take its tool on hearing and on auditory processing. With limits on speed and power nowhere in sight, these developments are rightly a matter of grave concern.

During the last few decades we have witnessed great technological developments and achievements, but we have also had to contend with the exponential increase in noise levels well beyond comfort level. The dramatic increase in environmental noise levels has awakened a renewed interest in the problem of noise pollution and its effect on health and well being of not only adults, but our children as well.

It has been noted that with increasing noise, changes do occur in brain chemistry. When this occurs in the workplace, the effect is predictably low productivity, a marked increase in accident rates on the job, and a deterioration in the quality of life usually compounded with high frequency hearing loss.

There is reason to believe that our children are also affected in very subtle ways by the unrestrained effects of environmental noise pollution. Dramatic alterations in thought processes of children brought on by the constant and indiscriminate exposure to noise in their environment is evident. One 17-year old girl recently reported at our clinic that about two weeks earlier she attended a week-end party where the noise was excessive. At one point she had inadvertently moved closer to one of the speakers in the room, whereupon she was struck by a blast of noise that caused immediate pain and discomfort. She said her ears have not stop ringing since.

A parent I have recently encountered, said that her child frequently covers his ears in response to noise in the environment, noise that very often has little effect on her, but quite a profound effect on her child. In one instance a mother whose 6-year old son's hearing had just been tested and found perfectly normal, asked if we could supply her with a pair of earplugs for her son. She said that then she could take him to the cinema where he could enjoy some entertainment without having to cover his ears complaining that the noise was too loud.

Certainly no rational person is advocating an environment of silence. Complete silence in our environment is unreal, threatening and unnatural. We need sound for our physiological and psychological equilibrium. But it is the indiscriminate excess of noise that is worrisome and most disturbing. And by noise I mean anything that is superfluous, unwanted, random or disturbing in the environment, especially in the learning environment, namely the classroom.

Noise as a contributor

Educators are now beginning to take a more critical look at the problem of excessive classroom noise. There is reason to believe that noise is having a profound affect on the psychological and physiological well—being of many of our children in the classroom. This finely tuned mechanism, known as auditory processing, is insidiously being rendered incapable of creative function by the encroachment of persistent noise within the learning environment. Learning is being modified in ways not clearly understood, due mainly to the effect of noise on the thinking processes of children especially those who already have processing difficulties. These children are having great difficulty with sequencing of information, showing marked deficits in language and cognitive functioning, especially when analytical and complex tasks are demanded in the presence of noise.

In the noisy classroom, the child's ability to process information is greatly compromised. Especially when at times in the classroom noise can reach the level where learning can be severely disrupted. What changes occur in the auditory perception of the child due to the persistent bombardment of noise have not been clearly documented. However, what has been determined is that the child with auditory perceptual difficulties functions poorly at all times, or at times ceases to function at all in the presence of interfering background noise.

Most of these children are of normal intelligence, with no visible signs of emotional disturbance, but they seem to have unusual difficulty organizing an appropriate response to incoming information when noise is present in their environment. Their organizing, storage and retrieval capacity of information for immediate use show diminished capacity. Because the incoming information is indecipherable, the child finds it difficult to attach meaning to what he hears so that he cannot make maxim use of it for academic purposes. This child will have difficulty surviving in the regular classroom as they struggle to keep pace with teacher and peers. On the other hand when placed in a noise free environment this child is far more focused and productive.

As has been mentioned earlier many factors may interfere with the normal influx of impulses to the brain for processing. Factor such as noise, is by far a major contributor. What happens in the classroom is that as noise levels increase, meaningful dialogue between teacher and student decreases. In this busy noisy environment the teacher strives to maintain some semblance of order and discipline. This is usually impossible to achieve under such conditions. One mother said that when her son is placed in such situations, he ceases to function altogether. He has been moved around the classroom several times to improve his concentration, but to no avail. On the other hand, when he is given individualized instruction in quiet he is far more focused and productive.

The reason the child functions poorly in noise is because of something called psycho-acoustical masking which interferes with communication in a dramatic way. Psycho-acoustical masking occurs when incoming noise alters the quality of speech communication. Though this noise may not be loud enough to cause a hearing disorder, it is nevertheless intense and persistent enough to interfere with speech communication to the extent where it raises the threshold for speech to a level, if intense enough can distort the quality of the message until it is unintelligible or at times inaudible. As the signal(speech) distorts, it becomes more and more difficult for the child to decipher the message for decoding by the brain.

Furthermore, doubling the distance between teacher and child reduces further the intensity of the signal from the teacher to the child by a factor of four. Therefore, when the teacher is busy attending to the varied needs of every pupil in that large noisy classroom, every time she distances herself from the child trying to communicate with her, the intensity of the signal is reduced by four or even sixteen depending on how far it must travel before reaching the child's ear.

When this is coupled with the extraneous noise coming from outside the classroom walls, the masking effect is increased exponentially as intelligibility of the message is decreased proportionately. Then, when you add to this other factors such as the presentation of information by the teacher, her style of presentation, material presented, room acoustics and a wide range of factors compounding how effectively the message will or will not be delivered to the child for processing, one can see the level of challenge a child is presented with on a daily basis.

As these conditions make it increasingly difficult for normal processing of information to take place at the cortical level, many children just simply give up and cease to function, much to the chagrin of the teacher. Some children just become totally detached. The teacher's yelling and threatening the child to gain his attention only aggravates the situation by increasing noise levels. If and when the teacher manages to establish order by raising her voice above the level of the ambient noise in the classroom, unfortunately, he has already missed substantial portions of the information so that there are too many gaps in the message to make sense of what he now hears.

The alert classroom teacher therefore should always be aware of the point where attention in the classroom has been compromised. The struggle to survive in the classroom is real. One parent told me that sometimes her child comes home form school, drops his books on the table, holds his head between his hands and cries: "O mother, that classroom noise . . . that awful noise!" What is more frustrating is that the child's poor performance often leads authorities to conclude that he is lazy or of low intelligence and thus apply undue pressure on him to perform.

Auditory processing disorder

When does auditory processing become a disorder? Experts agree that an auditory processing disorder is the inability to utilize incoming information in a normal manner due to some defect in the processing capabilities of the central auditory nervous system. A collapse of this kind causes a breakdown in any or all of the auditory abilities described thus far. The child hears normally but there is an inappropriate use of information received. This eventually leads to characteristics patterns of behavior typically displayed in children with auditory processing deficits. When such behavior becomes significant enough to interfere with the child's ability to perform academically or even socially, he or she is said to have a perceptual disorder.

In most cases one distinct behavioral characteristic is a deficit in auditory comprehension. Noticeably the child may display a tendency for random "fading in" and "fading out" of understanding things. This is referred to at times as intermittent auditory imperceptions. In some cases this is misinterpreted by parents and teachers as a hearing loss, missing certain portions of a message presented, while only responding to other parts of the message, but in reality it is not.

This subaverage performance in academics, eventually generates a feeling of insecurity and inadequacy in the child and lays the foundation for changes in personality behavior. Not willing to express himself by word of mouth for fear of ridicule, the child gradually avoids verbal communication as much as he can. In the classroom he struggles for self-identity. In his struggle there may be moments of irritability, isolation, frustration and at times even aggression. This child's learning experience is not a pleasant one. He is indeed lost in the classroom.

Chapter 9

The Causes of Central Auditory Processing Disorders (CAPD)

Although the precise cause or causes of *central auditory processing disorders* (CAPD) are still not clearly understood, it is recognized as distinct from attention deficiency disorder (ADD), or attention deficiency/hyperactivity disorder (ADHD), and dyslexia. ADD/ADHD is a pathologic condition or syndrome characterized by inattentiveness, distractibility, impulsiveness, and hyperactivity, which may require prescribed medication to reduce the level of hyperactivity, so that learning can take place. Dyslexia is an interneurosensory learning disability characterized by the ability to learn the spoken word and recognize what letters look like, and an inability to associate the images with the way they sound for reading purposes.

CAPD is a separate condition with its own idiosyncratic characteristics. These characteristics are significant enough to inhibit learning and influence all aspects of auditory functioning, both verbal and nonverbal. One theory attributes the condition to differences in the way the brain is wired for sound and to poor interconnections among the neural circuits supporting language so that incoming auditory stimuli are not properly routed to their appropriate designations for processing. As a result, children with CAPD respond inconsistently to sound and are sometimes regarded as hearing impaired.

Since the brain is poorly "wired" for language, and its circuits are badly interconnected, the language skills of these children are noticeably affected. The result is poor storage and retrieval of information, which is manifested by their inadequate receptive and expressive language performance. Also evident is poor sequential ordering of the critical elements of speech sounds, which affect the ability to remember sounds in words and words in sentences in their sequential order for proper expression.

Disorders of the central auditory mechanism range from simple abnormal auditory behaviors due to a lack of proper environmental stimulation to severe forms of pathology due to some specific central lesion. A central disorder arising from some form of neurological disturbance may not only influence the child's ability to think but also affect other neural processes as well, causing a break down in all of the central auditory abilities described so far. For instance, a vascular accident, brain trauma, or a disease such as kernicterus can disrupt vital central processing mechanisms that alter the proper development and functioning of the CANS.

It must be stressed here, however, that perceptual disorders contributing to some form of *learning disability* is not necessarily due to brain damage. Children may be perceptually handicapped for a number of reasons not directly related to brain damage. For instance, blindness, deafness, and types of emotional disturbances referred to as perceptual are not all necessarily neurogenic in origin.

Early Intervention

When a child is thought to have a CAPD, he or she should receive a thorough neurological, ophthalmological, and audiological evaluation before any form of management is contemplated, in order to rule out the possibility of a highly consequential medical disease. Neurological findings are of particular interest because they indicate the developmental status of the child's central auditory nervous system. Since the growth of language relates to the progressive maturation of the cerebral cortex, these findings have important implications for reading and language development.

Since it is estimated that 85 percent or more of our learning comes by way of the eyes (Martmer, 1959), it is imperative that children undergo a thorough eye examination as a part of the neurological work-up before they enter school, to furnish a basis for specialized treatment, if warranted, and to provide guidance regarding their educational needs. As a matter of interest, it is recommended that children whose eyes have not matured to the point of *accommodation* (the power of altering the focus of the eye readily for near objects) should not be subjected to the educational discipline of reading until appropriate measures have been implemented (Garrison and Force, 1965).

Audiologist, on the other hand, focuses on the auditory perceptual abilities and can assess them based on the child's ability to respond appropriately to auditory stimuli under different conditions of signal distortion and competition. If the child has CAPD, he or she will experience great difficulty executing certain auditory tasks during these tests procedures. The level of difficulty the child experiences while relying on a defective auditory channel is a measure of the dysfunction.

If there is no brain dysfunction of a medical nature that can be detected, educational approaches must be directed toward addressing those specific abnormal auditory behaviors that are affecting learning. These milder forms of impairment generally express themselves (in varying degrees of severity) in processing deficiency in auditory discrimination, language comprehension, auditory sequencing, and auditory memory. When intellectual deficiencies such as these exist, a child may still learn if given the proper educational guidance and environmental enrichment, reinforced with ample language and cognitive stimulation.

In most cases, the auditory deficiency, rather than being influenced by a specific medical lesion, is affected by an absence of adequate environmental stimulation and challenging conditions to which the child has been exposed over prolonged periods of time. Restricted forms of self-expression in some instances mirror the cultural milieu in which the child has been nurtured.

We know that input from the ear helps shape the auditory cortex into its permanent form by age four by which time the brain is hardwired for hearing. We also know the cortex is a constantly changing entity, powerfully shaped by experiences in childhood and throughout life. The message, therefore, is abundantly clear—expose the child to a profusion of appropriate environmental experiences once the child is developmentally ready for them, and learning will be facilitated. In the case of CAPD, although the brain may be poorly wired for language, the science of neuroplasticity teaches us that the brain is "massively plastic" and can be rewired or reprogrammed with the help of rigorous training and intensive cognitive stimulation so that these weak neural connections in the various parts supporting language can be eventually strengthened (Greenwald, 1999).

Therefore, once the child has been properly evaluated by specialized tests of central auditory skills and the specific disorder or disorders identified, then a deficit-specific program tailored to address the child's auditory needs can be undertaken. The end product of any habilitative strategy is to effect lasting and permanent change in the child's intellectual functioning. Ultimately, the child must learn to make good use of the information he or she receives through the auditory channel. When this is achieved, there will be an increased capacity for abstract thinking and reasoning displayed in the child's overall functional behavior through the efficient use of listening.

Cerebral Pathology Affecting Processing

While the causes of CAPD have not been definitively explained, certain features commonly characterize this condition. Bellis (1998) observes that

- there is a disruption or alteration in the continuous flow of information on its way to the brain that is not attributed to hearing loss, though hearing loss may significantly contribute to the problem. For this reason, a hearing loss is generally ruled out as a variable before testing for CAPD begins.
- this disruption has an adverse affect on phonetic as well as linguistic information from the time the ear received it to the time the brain attributes meaning to it. Why central auditory processing disorders affect speech and language the way it does is not clearly understood except that there is a logical connection between how a child hears and how he or she speaks—a dysfunction in one area is bound to create a dysfunction in the other.

- CAPD can occur for different reasons and assume different forms, each of which negatively impacts on the child's ability to learn.
- CAPD can occur at various stages of the child's central nervous system (CNS) development, affecting language development, and intellectual and social skills.

In order for an individual to perform certain auditory tasks, such as dichotic listening (presenting two messages to both ears simultaneously, but with both messages being different), the two cerebral hemispheres of the brain, left and right, must be able to communicate effectively. Note the slightly larger left hemisphere in Figure 9.1 is generally dominant for language. To perform a dichotic task, the individual must synchronize listening tasks interdependently between both hemispheres. At times, there may be poor bilateral integration of the right and left hemispheres, causing both sides to work independently and out of synchrony with each other.

Figure 9.1.

The cerebral hemispheres—left and right cerebral hemispheres viewed form a superior aspect: (1) frontal pole (2) middle frontal gurus (3) superior frontal sulcus (4) superior frontal gyrus (5) interhemispheric fissure (6) precentral sulcus (7) precentral gyrus (8) central sulcus (9) postcentral gyrus (10) postcentral sulcus (11) superior parietal lobule (12) occipital gyri (13) occipital pole

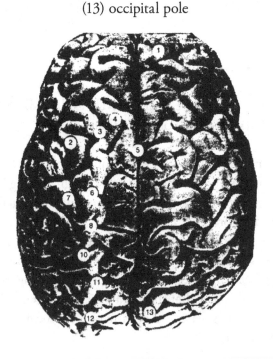

At other times, there may be inadequate specialization of the hemispheres, causing poor auditory—visual—spatial difficulties. All these problems have the cumulative effect of creating uncoordinated sensory activity in the brain. Furthermore, any disorder, especially in the posterior portion of the corpus callosum, significantly affects the efficient transfer of auditory information across the brain from one hemisphere to the other. Those disorders that affect the function of the brain and do not allow the two hemispheres to communicate efficiently may be influenced by a deficiency in the following cerebral areas (shown in Figure 9.2)—Broca's area (44 and 45), visual—auditory association area (37), angular gyrus area (39), Wernike's auditory association cortex area (22, 39, and 40), and Heschl's gyrus (41, 42).

Figure 9.2.

Language areas—Cytoarchitectural division of the areas related to language: (22) auditory; association area (37); visual—auditory association area (39), angular gurus (41 and 42), Heschl's gyrus (44 and 45), Broca's area (22, 39, and 40), Wernicke's area (xxx) area traditionally related to writing

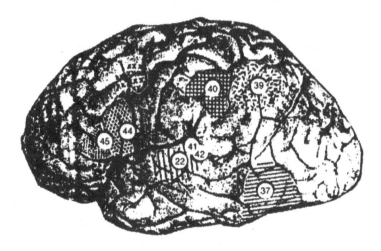

Corpus Callosum

The corpus callosum not shown is a fibrous bundle of axons three hundred million, forming a bridge between the brain's two hemispheres. These fibers connect the right and left hemispheres of the cerebral cortex and are primarily responsible for the communication and integration of information from the two hemispheres of the brain. The left hemisphere of the brain is dominant for such functions as follows:

- speech and language function
- temporal ordering
- reading and writing
- concrete reasoning
- analyzing
- sequencing of auditory stimuli

The right hemisphere of the brain is dominant for the following:

- music perception
- acoustic contours-stress and rhythm and intonation of speech
- the emotional element of speech
- spatial and artistic relationships
- figure and facial recognition
- gestalt perception

It is of importance to recognize cerebral hemispheric dominance since marked deviations between verbal and nonverbal learning often indicate in which hemisphere a dysfunction resides. The neurology of verbal behavior differs from that of nonverbal behavior. For instance, verbal abilities are generally localized in the left (dominant) hemisphere of the brain and are typically responsible for verbal function, while nonverbal tasks are localized in the right hemisphere of the brain and are more diffused in the brain than verbal abilities.

In the 1960s, when testing dichotic listening tasks in normal right-handed children, researchers found that scores in the right ear were consistently higher than scores in the left ear (Bryden, 1963; Dirks, 1964; Kimura, 1961a; Satz, Achenback, Pattishall, and Fennell, 1965). This phenomenon later became known as *the Right Ear Advantage* (REA) in normal right-handed listeners. It was noted, however, that this REA disappeared with neuromaturation of the system as the child grew older; with the passage of time, scores reflected more of an adult performance and the disparity between ears disappeared. A child experiencing CAPD, however, tends to persist with *right ear advantage* long after the system should have reached maturity.

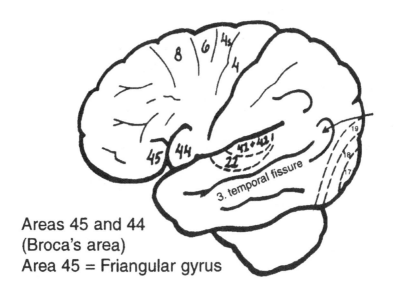

Areas 45 and 44
(Broca's area)
Area 45 = Friangular gyrus

Left Frontal Lobe (Broca's Speech Area)

A disorder that is confined to the left frontal lobe, known as Broca's area (areas 44 and 45), will result in difficulty executing speech when the dominant hemisphere is involved. This is referred to as *Broca's aphasia*. The memory engrams here connected with speech are affected while comprehension of the spoken language remains largely intact. The individual knows what he or she wants to say, but speech is difficult to execute, even though the vocal musculature for speech is not paralyzed. In children, however, because of the plasticity of the brain with a disorder in this area the child can be taught to speak by utilizing the nondominant cerebral hemisphere of the brain when the dominant hemisphere is impaired.

Temporal—Occipital—Parietal Region (Angular Gyrus)

Disorders in the dominant cerebral hemisphere of the temporal—occipital—parietal area, known as the angular gyrus (area 39), result in a condition known as *visual aphasia*—also known as *word blindness*, or *alexia* and *agraphia*; in other words, they cause an inability to read and write. Individuals see the printed words but cannot read them because such symbols are meaningless to them. It is like looking at Arabic or Chinese writing. All the untrained eye sees are the characters and the curved lines, but the person cannot read them because they have no specific meaning and representation for someone not familiar with the language.

Wernicke's Area (the Phonemic Zone)

Damage on the dominant side in a right-handed person results in the individual being able to hear but unable to understand what is being said. Unlike in Broca's aphasia, where the person understands the spoken word but cannot execute speech, individuals can speak and hear the spoken word but are unable to comprehend what is being said. They speak but make mistakes unknowingly owing to their inability to monitor their language and understand their own words. Such individuals experience sound without any meaning. This is referred to as *Wernicke's aphasia* or *word deafness* (even though the person is not actually deaf). At times, a patient may have a cerebral artery stroke and may display characteristics of both Broca's and Wernicke's aphasia, a condition known as *mixed aphasia*.

Heschl's Gyrus

Finally, a disorder in *Heschl's gyrus* the area (41 and 42) in the dominant hemisphere, known as the *auditory reception area*, also affects the ability of the individual to understand the spoken word. This is also known as *word deafness*. As in Wernicke's aphasia the patient isn't deaf; he or she hears but cannot understand what is said.

Summary

There are certain disorders that affect the function of the brain and prevent the two hemispheres from communicating efficiently. This affects an individual's ability to perform certain communication tasks, such as dichotic listening. Such dysfunctions may be located in the following areas of the brain:

- the corpus callosum
- Broca's area
- Angular gurus
- Wernike's area (the phonemic zone)
- Heschl's gurus (primary auditory reception region)
- Visual—auditory association area

Dysfunctions of these areas disturb perception and reduce children's total learning experience. It is crucial, therefore, that when children are suspected of central auditory processing disorders that they be given a thorough neurological, audiological, and opthamological evaluation to ascertain the status of the central nervous system whose development has important implications for the development of language and learning.

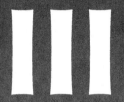

PART

III

MANAGEMENT

Chapter 10

Help Is Available

The problem with children experiencing CAPD is that they do not possess the capacity to manage information effectively. Because the incoming information is not properly organized, it is as though they had no information at all. Their difficulty is learning through a defective auditory channel. As mentioned in the previous chapters, something intercepts information from the ear on its way to the brain for interpretation. This disconnection results in enormous difficulty with translating sound into language, which severely undermines the child's overall language processing capabilities. Much academic learning is auditory or visual or both and a child may have deficiencies in either or both of these areas. Before the child can be helped, it is crucial to know which input channels are not in tact and how they can be enhanced by training.

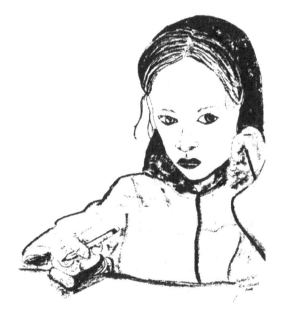

Something intercepts information on its way to the brain.

Management of the problems of children with listening disorders such as CAPD is based on the theory of *neuroplasticity of the brain*. Because of its plasticity, the brain can undergo organizational change as a result of synaptic activity that is critical to *learning* and *memory* (Greenwald, 1999; Hebb, 1949). The reactive brain has the ability to grow with use and decreases with disuse.

Plasticity implies that the structure of the brain, with its highly complex *cytoarchitecture*, can change and is constantly changing, shaped by our experiences and ongoing activity throughout life. It is known that the central auditory nervous system (CANS) itself is not predetermined and unalterably fixed but can and does alter its "neural wiring" throughout *a* person's *lifetime.* In other words, it is not rigidly preprogrammed.

Change can be achieved through intensive training by the repeated use of the *synapse* (point or junction at which nerve impulses move from one neuron to the other to convey information). This requires constant repetition of stimuli until a desired pattern is established (Aoki and Siekevitz, 1988; Rauschecker and Marler, 1987). Thus the brain can be reprogrammed to function efficiently and to bring about the desired permanent organizational change in behavior.

Any management strategy for children with auditory problems mentioned above, therefore, has to increase the efficiency of the processing of information by the central nervous system and thereby modify dysfunction influencing the learning process. This requires a team approach among a number of professionals since no one person can be expected to have competencies in all the different areas of central auditory function. Only specialists in the various aspects of the child's health can put together a composite picture of this child's needs and formulate flexible approaches and solutions that meet the child's specific requirements. The goal of the management team is to offer a unified, educational, and balanced approach to the management profile.

The Child's Profile

The management protocol for the child must be deficit-specific, with the goal of raising the efficiency in proportion to the child's strengths so that more uniform abilities are achieved. By this I mean, the child has both strengths and weaknesses—low points in his abilities. Every effort must be made to strengthen those areas of deficiency in proportion to his strengths. Let us assume a child is not a visual learner, but is a strong auditory learner. Some educators would advocate capitalizing on the auditory approach to the neglect of the visual, hoping that he would generalize the auditory facility to all other areas of function. This may be so with the normal learner, but children with learning disabilities are not capable of doing this, and that is what sets them apart from the normal learner. Consequently, any diagnosis, evaluation, and management of the child must consider the matrix of variables that will ultimately shape this child's future.

Moreover, any management strategy must begin with more than a mere diagnosis of this child's present condition; it must also look into the developmental history of the child's difficulties.

Therefore, before recommendations for management can be implemented, a *profile* of the child is needed. The compiling of a profile is an attempt to generate information about the child's past and present functional behavior, his or her levels of functioning, intellectual growth and capacity, perceptual development, levels of conceptualization, motor coordination, visual and auditory abilities, social maturity and emotional and psychological adjustment, along with other abilities and characteristics that are inherent potentialities for development. In other words, a profile should reflect a thorough knowledge of the whole child.

As was mentioned earlier, there are no blanket recommendations for children with CAPD since the problem has many dimensions, affecting emotional, physical, psychological, and intellectual performance. Because of the wide range of differences between children, one must avoid generalization and oversimplification. Some management strategies will concentrate on securing focused attention, others on preventing of distractibility, others the control of proximity (e.g., closer to the teacher, more distance from peers), and yet others, on the rate and manipulation of verbal and nonverbal behavior. In other words, different approaches should be used to accommodate the specific educational needs of the child.

To prepare the profile, a competent personal must first examine the child in terms of his or her special communication needs and the listening and learning environment in which he or she is asked to function daily. In the process, they must determine the kind of placement that is most appropriate given the child's particular needs (*selective placement*). The most logical place to start with such an assessment is, of course, in the classroom. The assessment should focus on those aspects of the setting and material delivery that facilitate or impede the child's learning progress. Certain questions in particular should be addressed before any recommendations are made. They are as follows:

Setting

- Where is the teaching to take place?
- Is auditory attention helped or distracted by other stimuli auditory or visual?
- What is the child's ability to function in the present classroom setting? What are the difficulties currently encountered?
- How well does the child perform under different listening or learning situations?
- Does the child have the capacity to cope in this particular classroom?
- What are the child's minimum survival skills in the present setting?
- Is the child able to pay auditory attention and can he or she sustain it over reasonable periods of time?
- Is the child able to follow aural information (tracking) within this setting?

- What is this child's ability to follow directions?

Conditions of presentation

- *Maximize attention:* How can the presentation of information be adjusted to maximize attention, cooperation, and performance from this child and at the same time minimize distraction?
- *Teaching methodology and style of teaching:* What is the most effective teaching approach for this child?
- *Classroom acoustics:* How noisy is the current environment and what effect does it have on this child's ability to perform? What simple alterations can be made in the classroom to improve acoustics and, hence, listening?
- *Learning situations:* What types of learning situations will the child be generally exposed to?
- *Demands:* What are the seating arrangements? What is the curriculum? What is demanded of the child in general?
- *Availability of assistive listening devices (ALD):* Would assistive listening devices help or impede processing/

Once assessment is made, the management team involved in the habilitation of the child _must now_ address all of the above concerns as they formulate a management protocol that accommodates the child's auditory needs. This team is likely to consist among others of the following:

- educational audiologist
- speech—language pathologist
- educational psychologist
- educator or teacher
- caregiver

Roles of Management Team Members

Educational Audiologist

Educational audiologists assess the auditory perceptual abilities of children through screening and diagnostic hearing tests. They monitor those who are at risk for processing difficulties and those classified as hearing impaired. As has been mentioned earlier, their assessment of processing difficulties is based on the child's ability to respond appropriately to auditory stimuli under different conditions of signal distortion and competition. The rationale for this strategy is that a normal listener can tolerate mild distortion of speech stimuli and still process it, while a listener experiencing processing difficulties encounters severe problems with distorted speech due to the additional internal distortion that a defective mechanism generates.

Educational audiologists provide recommendations regarding auditory management strategies. They administer tests to assess different processes and different levels so that a specific processing disorder that affects the child's ability to learn can be identified. In cases where a deficiency is uncovered, they recommend management protocols to assist the child in overcoming the deficiency so that he can actualize his potential as a functional and productive part of the learning community.

The results of the audiological evaluation must be interpreted in terms of the implications they have on the child's functional behavior both in terms of his or her academic performance and social interaction. This step is known as the *process of demystification*. The interpretation of results for auditory processing dysfunction is one of the most critical tasks of educational audiologists. Great skill is required of the audiologist to translate his or her findings into practical terms that others can understand and implement, expressing clearly to what degree the disorder is affecting the child's ability to function.

Moreover, it is usually the educational audiologists who make decisions regarding the acoustical environment in which the child functions. The goal is to help the child get the most from classroom acoustics through simple strategic modifications. Such modifications must ultimately enhance the child's comprehension, and thereby contribute to the easy accessibility of information in the least acoustically competitive environment.

When necessary, audiologists also advise the school administrator or personnel regarding the selection of classroom educational amplification systems. The assistive listening devices recommended by the audiologist and used in the classroom to improve listening are designed to maximize the teacher's ability to reach the child's ear under all likely listening conditions. These devices are used so that teachers do not have to raise their voice to get the child's attention. They mildly amplify the teacher's voice above the level of background noise present in the classroom. Whatever amplification system is used to be effective it must

- provide ample audibility and clarity of speech reaching the child's ear
- improve teacher—child communication without the teacher having to change the teaching style significantly
- be simple enough to use (mobile and comfortable to wear—be durable)
- be free from acoustical and electrical interferences
- accommodate a whole range of teaching arrangements
- provide flexibility

Audiologists also make suggestions for enhancing speech intelligibility in the classroom.

These suggestions include

- reducing the level of background noise and *reverberation time* in the classroom
- reducing the distance between teacher and the child to enhance speech intelligibility

Reverberation Time

Reverberation is the prolongation of sound emanating from its source and is the most important factor when considering the acoustical qualities of a room. *Reverberation time* is the time required for a sound to decrease by 60 bB in a room after its source has stopped. Optimum reverberation time should not exceed half a second. This criterion is generally not met in most of today's classrooms. Frequently, the poor acoustic conditions existing in the classroom create sound reflections that cause a part of the signal to persist longer than the time required for the ear to respond to it. Classrooms that are small, rectangular in shape, and have smooth wall surfaces produce a high level of reverberation.

What makes reverberation increasingly difficult for the child is that there are two waves present. There is the direct wave, that part of the signal that goes directly to the ear of the listener, and the indirect wave, that part of the wave that travels by an indirect route to the listener's ear after bouncing off smooth surfaces. Speech in a highly reverberant environment such as this is subject to a high level of distortion. The weak consonant sounds are the first to be distorted due to the masking affect of the noise on these low-intensity speech sounds.

Sound frequencies are analyzed by the basilar membrane located in the inner ear. To analyze pitch properly, this membrane must be heavily damped (have decreased vibration). When the membrane is not properly damped, overwriting (one response on top of another) occurs, resulting in signal distortion, and such is the case with consonant sounds in noise.

Figure 9.1
Basilar membrane:
A membrane in the inner ear responsible for analysis of pitch.

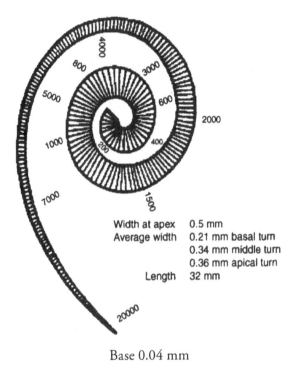

Width at apex   0.5 mm
Average width   0.21 mm basal turn
                 0.34 mm middle turn
                 0.36 mm apical turn
Length   32 mm

Base 0.04 mm

Environments with a lot of noise and reverberation make listening extra difficult for children with auditory processing difficulties. First, the direct signal arrives already distorted by noise. Soon afterward, the indirect signal arrives after bouncing off the smooth surfaces in the classroom. A noisy environment with poor acoustics makes listening extremely difficult for children who are already experiencing language and speech difficulties because of poor decoding speech capabilities. Reverberation can be reduced in a number of ways—*some of these methods will be discussed in later.*

Distance

When the distance between the speaker (teacher) and the listener (child) is increased the intensity of the speech signal is reduced. This problem can be minimized through *preferential seating*—a seating arrangement in which children who have problems with hearing or processing information sit closer to the teacher. Preferential seating means that the child can easily follow the teacher in the classroom, which increases his or her ability to concentrate on other processing tasks. The use of *ALDs* or other sound field educational amplification systems can also help minimize the problem of distance.

Speech—Language Pathologist

Speech—language pathologists are directly involved in the implementation of language-based therapeutic techniques and interventions. They may also be involved in the testing of the CAPD child since they possess tools that can assess the auditory perceptual abilities of children with CAPD. Speech—language pathologists are likely to carry out many of the management suggestions made following a comprehensive central auditory assessment by the educational audiologist. In short, they work closely with the audiologist to develop and to implement management recommendations and strategies that will enhance the child's listening capabilities in the classroom.

Educational Psychologist

If listening problems are identified, psychological counseling may be recommended. Educational psychologists can test children to determine to what degree their auditory problems are affecting their ability to learn, and they outline the consequences of the emotional disturbances that processing problems may be causing. A child may well be experiencing continued symptoms of frustration and depression due to the continual academic struggle or failure he is having. Psychologists are an important resource in dealing with children having such difficulties, providing valuable information regarding the social—emotional impact of the disorder and its effects on the cognitive functioning of the child. Indeed, many children who come for central auditory processing assessment may have already been seen by an educational psychologist for a psychological evaluation.

Educator

Everyone involved in the teaching of a child with CAPD must know that the special educational needs of the child have to be met if he or she is to attain full academic potential. Many well-intentioned teachers want to help the child learn, but they feel inadequate or unprepared to cope with the special educational needs associated with CAPD. In addition, the classroom teacher is always limited by the constraints of time. In general, what is the attitude of the teacher with regard to children with CAPD? The way many teachers see it is that they are already overwhelmed by the individual demands and needs of a classroom full of children so they have limited time left for coping with yet another problem about which they have little or no knowledge.

It is not uncommon to hear the teacher remark about children with CAPD that they do not try hard enough or that they never pay attention. These children are often described as having difficulty following multistep directions, and in completing tasks. They are said to be withdrawn, sullen, and antisocial never wanting to participate in classroom activity. They never seem to understand what is said and respond inappropriately to the discussion at hand. They frequently ask to have things repeated. Teachers also frequently complain about their poor spelling, messy and hard to decipher handwriting, and inattentiveness. Such remarks reflect a general lack of understanding of the child's auditory confusion.

It is the task of educators to provide the basic skills for the child to survive not only within the classroom, but outside the classroom as well. The skills that are most essential are reading, writing and reasoning. At the same time there are many complex forces present within the classroom environment which interact to impede the development of these vital skills. These forces create a barrier between the child and his aspirations to learn. If these obstacles are not minimized or indeed eliminated altogether, he may never achieve full intellectual prowess.

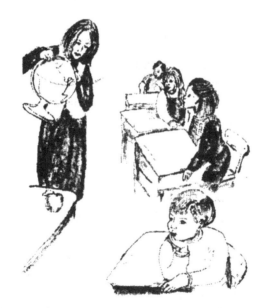

The child is often described as withdrawn, sullen, antisocial,
never participating in classroom activity.

Teachers need not be unduly perturbed by the presence of a child with CAPD in the classroom. What they need to do is follow a few simple strategies that constitute the minimal requirements to achieve teaching success with such children. In fact, most of the strategies suggested for improved listening and learning for children with CAPD or with poor listening skills can be of benefit to every listening child in the classroom. The necessary modifications can be implemented with the least amount of alteration to teaching style and with no additional time and effort expended on the part of the teacher.

To be successful in teaching the child with listening and processing disorders, teachers should have a basic understanding of such teaching principles as motivation, reinforcement, and reward. A teacher who is able to use these strategies effectively will observe marked success in the classroom with children having processing difficulties. When these strategies are properly implemented, the classroom can become less of a threat to the child and more of a place of challenge where cognitive, linguistic, and academic skills are nurtured.

Teachers must keep in mind that whether or not they are inclined to confront the issue sooner or later they will inevitably encounter children with CAPD in their classroom and will be forced to make decisions regarding their learning. The challenge for teachers, therefore, is to make sure that these children are given the opportunity to develop in harmony with their potentialities and that the necessary educational provisions are available for their success.

Caregiver

Studies have shown that when applied very early in life, family-centered intervention is highly successful in terms of productivity, permanence, and practicality. The forces that nurture, sustain, and shape the child's communicative development early on have an enduring effect on the child for life (Bronfenbrenner, 1974).

The importance of caregivers' active participation in stimulating the language processing capabilities of their children cannot be overemphasized; in particular, the mother's involvement during the child's prelinguistic period of development is absolutely crucial. The caregiver's natural ability to respond to and stimulate and interact with the child during the early years is fundamental to the development of good cognitive skills, which permanently influence the child's linguistic, intellectual, emotional and social growth throughout life. Substantial evidence indicates that children who have been deprived of parental interaction and were neglected by caregivers manifest significant developmental delays in all aspects of growth and development when compared to those children who have received it during the prelinguistic period of development (Blager and Martin, 1976; Cicchetti and Beeghly, 1987; Fox et al., 1988; Hughes and Dibrezzo, 1987; McCauley and Swisher, 1987).

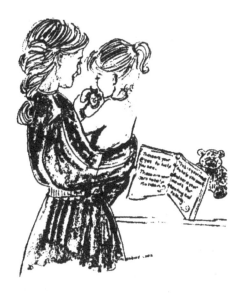

Parental interaction with the child is crucial to the development
of language and cognitive skills.

Children with CAPD need the support of everyone, especially their caregivers, to cope with the difficulties they experience as they try to gain the acceptance and approval of adults and peers. Caregivers may become frustrated and impatient at the slow pace of their children's progress. It is important to remember that often children who may be regarded as slow and unintelligent may in reality be suffering from serious emotional maladjustment difficulties, which are actually masking their true mental abilities and potential. Therefore, as understandable as it may be, impatience on the part of the caregiver can be self-defeating and may only lead to further damage to the child's sense of personal worth. It often has the effect of limiting the growth of these children's exploratory behavior, creativity, and self-confidence.

Undoubted, children having processing difficulties manage information slowly—more slowly than their peers—but, nevertheless, they processes it just the same, only at a slower rate. When they succeed, caregivers should bolster their ego and personal worth with praise and reinforcement. These children need to succeed in tasks regarded by themselves and others as worthwhile. Thus they are best served if caregivers recognize their limitations and strengths and accept them as they are while encouraging their efforts to solve problems within their grasp.

It is important to keep in mind that the situation is frustrating for them as well. They feel that they will never be able to attain their full potential and live up to their caregivers' expectations. Such feelings of inadequacy are often counterproductive and lead to bouts of guilt and defeatism on the part of the child. It is better for caregivers to interact positively in the child's day-to-day activities and encourage progress, rather than constantly emphasize their shortcomings. Caregivers should show that they care and understand what the child is going through. This keeps the child from feeling isolated, reduces his or her frustration level, and alleviates feelings of helplessness and inadequacy.

An emotionally insecure child is a lonely child, with self-confidence thoroughly eroded by persistent cycles of failure. These feelings of failure and inadequacy are marks of a weak ego, which breeds insecurity and low self-esteem or, conversely, highly aggressive and hostile behavior. This form of emotional immaturity has a tendency to invariably project into human relationships, causing maladjustment and withdrawal from social participation. Groups of frustrated youth may eventually become social isolates, resorting to drugs and other forms of deviant behavior as a solution to their problems and eventually direct their hostility toward institutions they see as symbols of society working against them.

Although all caregivers may not be able to spend as much time as required with their children as home educators, the most constant and influential teacher of the child is still the caregiver. Caregivers should assist their children at home as much as possible, especially when it comes to reading activities and other academic pursuits, helping them compensate for what they might have missed during the noisy classroom sessions of the day. This one-on-one tutoring at home assists the caregivers in mapping the child's daily achievements and charting his or her overall progress.

In terms of charting progress, caregivers must work cooperatively with other team members assisting the child so that progress can be better documented. Both caregivers and professional are indispensable in reinforcing techniques for language acquisition and facilitating the transfer of information from the classroom to everyday life situations. Carry-over activities from the classroom to the home can strongly reinforce what the child has accomplished during the school sessions. While doing household chores, for example, caregivers should talk constantly to the child about what they are doing, especially if the child is not particularly expressive.

Caregivers who want their children to be expressive should make use of every opportunity to improve their children's speech by motivating them to talk and get satisfaction and enjoyment from talking. One method is to do a lot of naming and observation while engaging with them in activities, with the aim of associating sound with experiences. This can involve making games out of naming objects, animals, and pictures in books and identifying objects while driving. As much as possible, it is useful to time auditory stimuli with the experience the child is having to reinforce the association.

Such techniques enrich children's vocabulary, expanding their receptive and expressive language proficiency. Soon speech might become an enjoyable experience, and children will begin looking out for opportunities to express themselves whenever they can. Frequent visits to the store, park, community events, and interesting places can all be transformed into pleasant everyday learning experiences.

It is evident that such interaction eventually goes beyond the development of the children's vocalization activity. It ultimately influences the development of their self-esteem, self-worth, and indeed emotional growth and social adjustment. In summary, the caregiver's role is crucial not merely in terms of language learning, but in terms of the child's total growth and intellectual development.

Chapter 11

Clinical Cases

The three cases discussed in this chapter demonstrate some of the difficulties that children with listening disorders experience daily both in and outside the classroom. Before proceeding further, it should be pointed out that single-study investigations, such as case history reporting, make generalizations difficult. However, case history reporting does have its merit since among other things, it helps teachers and clinicians detect certain differences that set a child apart from the other children of the same age or maturity level in a group. Such observations help professionals in adapting methods and strategies to those characteristics of the child being studied. The case study approach is indispensable in tailoring specific therapies for the difficulties that a particular child's may be encountering.

Each case presented contains a list of management suggestions. As mentioned earlier, there are no blanket recommendations for children with CAPD; each child must be assessed individually, and a specific plan tailored to his or her individual needs must be developed. Consequently, the suggestions included here should serve only as guidelines for implementing approaches for a particular listening problem.

Case No. 1

Mary was seen at the audiology clinic for a comprehensive central auditory processing (CAP) assessment. Background information highlighted difficulty remaining focused on given tasks, with poor understanding of speech in less than ideal listening conditions. When spoken to, Mary often needed to have things repeated. Her mother was concerned that she did not interpret or recall incoming information accurately. However, she normally performed well under ideal, noise-free listening conditions, where her performance improved significantly as she became more focused and productive.

Mary showed poor listening skills, short memory span, and a high degree of inattentiveness in the classroom. These were worsened by Mary's low tolerance for background noise interference. In the presence of noise, she appeared less focused and responded only to parts of information presented. This behavior reduced her ability to process information accurately in class, requiring additional time and patience to figure out what was required. Mary insisted on understanding every detail of the information presented and become frustrated when unable to do so. This increased the delay time in processing information so that she was not able to keep pace with her peers, which frustrated her even more.

Mary's inability to properly interpret information was likely responsible for inappropriate psychosocial behavior, creating feelings of inadequacy and low self-esteem. Failure, frustration, and low self-confidence contributed to bouts of discouragement, making her emotionally sensitive, easily hurt, and frequently sullen and withdrawn. Occasionally, she became so anxious that she did not always repeat with accuracy what she heard. She consequently gave up, feeling that the task was too difficult for her to cope with.

Audiometric Test Results

Pure tone audiometry revealed normal hearing bilaterally. Speech audiometry was consistent with pure tone results and was normal in both ears, with speech recognition scores of 100 percent in the left ear and 96 percent in the right ear.

Observation and Conclusion

Based on normal findings of audiometric test results, a comprehensive CAP evaluation was initiated. Mary responded well to the test procedure. She exhibited a deficiency in the process of *auditory closure* that appears to fit the profile of an *auditory decoding deficit*.

Auditory Closure

Auditory decoding plays an important role in everyday listening activities in the classroom, and if affected, causes a disturbance in attention span and the ability to properly receive and interpret information as listening conditions deteriorate. Ordinarily, children seldom listen in ideal conditions in the classroom, anyway, and must daily contend with background noise, regional dialects, conversational partners who speak quietly or have bad diction and many other adverse factors that degrade information and increase communication difficulty. Not being able to rely on *closure skills* compounds the problem immensely.

Auditory closure is the ability of the brain to perceive the whole message even though parts of the message are omitted or distorted due to interference. Because auditory closure deficit is a decoding problem, it reduces the child's phonemic ability, causing him or her to require frequent repetition and clarification before the components of information are properly deciphered and understood. The child consequently retains too little information because of a limited memory span, which causes him or her to easily forget what is said. This makes keeping pace with teacher and peers difficult and generates a high degree of anxiety and frustration.

To improve Mary's ability to effectively use auditory closure skills, management must included environmental modifications. The use of an FM device for educational purposes, for example, might be of great benefit in this case, as it would enhance clarity of information reaching Mary's ears in the classroom.

As well, Mary should be taught certain specific skills to help her cope with understanding speech in background noise. For one, she should receive phonemic auditory awareness training to help her develop accurate phonemic representation. She must also learn to take advantage of sound cues to track speech in noise to achieve understanding. Her listening skills have to be sharpened to the point where she uses them to the maximum, especially when listening under less than ideal conditions. Additional compensatory strategies may include methods of monitoring comprehension and identifying all difficult listening situations in which Mary finds herself on a daily basis.

Behavioral Characteristics of Children with Auditory Decoding Deficit

Children with this deficiency, such as Mary, typically do not take advantage of the abundance of informational cues inherent in a message to glean understanding. They usually

- cannot decipher the phonemic components of a message in noise, so message is easily misunderstood
- retain too little information when listening
- processes information slowly and inaccurately
- normally hear well under ideal listening conditions, but if the problem is severe enough, may have difficulty even in quiet conditions
- make errors in speech and speech discrimination misarticulating many words or mishearing words by hearing only pieces or fragments of sound (e.g., "thought" for "fought," "hip" for "ship," "skate" for "stake," p for b, etc.)
- have difficulty deciphering fine acoustic differences in sounds
- have problems with sound blending
- cannot distinguish between such speech sounds as: /p/ and /k/; /f/ and /th/, especially when listening in noise
- have difficulty learning different meanings of words
- show poor retention of phonemes
- have a short attention span
- say "Huh?," "What?," and "I don't understand" often
- experience difficulty with grammar, vocabulary, semantic skills, and words having multiple meanings so that parents and teachers think the child has hearing loss

Management Suggestions

Treatment must be specific to Mary's auditory processing needs for closure (decoding) purposes. Although each case must be assessed individually, in general, teachers and caregivers can use the following strategies with children who have an *auditory closure deficiency*:

- Environmental modifications such as preferential seating can improve access to auditory information. The child must be placed at all times in a position where he or she has easy access to information so that acquisition of information is effortless. Teacher's should adjust their teaching approaches to accommodate the child's needs, not the other way around.
- Reduction of background noise in the classroom, improves intelligibility of speech.
- Individualized instruction in subjects with significant thought content may be necessary.
- Building closure skills from phonemic to sentence level is important. A speech—language pathologist and a reading specialist are resource persons to call upon for assistance in these activities.
- All activities should begin with simple listening tasks and progress to complex ones; for example, distinguishing between gross sounds should come first, before listening to fine sound differences.
- The child must demonstrate mastery of one level of new information before moving on to the next level. The level of complexity should be at first reduced to the point where the child can interpret what he or she hears accurately, then the level of complexity should be raised gradually.
- If vocabulary is new or unfamiliar, the child may become lost when new material is presented. To avoid this, the child should be familiarized with new words before each presentation of new material. Vocabulary building is important since newly learned words strengthen comprehension. As soon as a word is understood in isolation, it should be introduced in context. Information presented verbally without enough contextual or visual cues as when talking to the blackboard or not facing the child when speaking must be avoided.
- Spoken word and experience must be carefully timed so that the child can make the exact association.
- The child requires extra visual cues such as facial expressions, pictures, or gestures to complement the listening task. The child should be encouraged to use such visual cues to improve understanding when listening, meaning that he or she must be taught how to look and listen to the speaker.

- Overlearning of skills through drill repetition to recognize the keywords of message may be necessary.
- Under difficult listening conditions, the redundancy of the message should be increased to make that message easier to understand.
- Preteaching of unfamiliar vocabulary when dealing with new concepts is helpful.
- Information may need to be repeated or rephrased for improved comprehension. Rephrasing makes information clearer and allows the child to fill in parts that he or she has missed the first time. However, rephrasing is good only when sufficient information is added to the message to clarify the original concept.
- Techniques to improve speech discrimination and listening should be employed. The child should be taught to comprehend speech under conditions of varying difficulty.
- The child's ability to hear differences in sounds must be improve.
- Phoneme training (phonics), sound blending, and discrimination drills improve retention of phonemes and helps child learn to develop accurate phonemic representation, increasing the ability to receive and decode acoustic messages.
- Instructions should be given verbally as well as written.
- Assistive listening devices improve intelligibility in classroom. FM units in the classroom have been shown to improve academic performance and attention because they enhance the signal reaching the child's ear, filtering out background noise.
- Vocabulary building improves skills for auditory closure and teaches the child to utilize contextual derivations to determine word meaning.
- Word association games are useful.
- Noise-tolerance techniques are helpful.

Noise—Tolerance Technique

Children with auditory decoding problems often find it difficult to concentrate on the teacher when noise is present. One specific strategy aimed at improving their listening skills is to purposefully expose them to controlled noise in order to increase their tolerance to it. With this method, part of the lesson should be given against a background of controlled levels of noise.

Controlled levels of noise are best used when teaching subjects that are less demanding on the children's concentration. This helps them cope when they are compelled to learn in less than ideal listening conditions. All activity is geared toward helping these children listen in situations most likely to be encountered in the highly variable environment of everyday living. But children should not be overwhelmed with all kinds of meaningless sound in the listening or learning environment. Random, purposeless sound is distracting and counterproductive to the development of listening skills. Similarly, the child's visual world should not be saturated with highly stimulating visual activity when they are expected to listen.

Educators can increase noise tolerance in the classroom by following these steps:

- Call the child's attention and have him or her listen for an extraneous noise.
- Gradual increase of background noise until a tolerance for stronger sound is achieved.
- Use background noise that is either recorded or available on the radio and that can be controlled.
- Present materials or sounds at intensities not disturbing at first.
- Continue this practice for some time until tolerance can gradually be achieved.
- During the presentation of background noise, the clinician should speak with ample intensity as he or she would use in conversation with children when a similar amount of noise is present

The following are some further tips on how to increase the level of difficulty:

- Vary the background noise from lesson to lesson, sound effects, instrumental music, vocal music, and dramatic readings (especially those having two or more people talking at the same time) can all help children develop selective listening skills.
- Use your judgment as to which part of the lesson to present against background distraction. The content of the distracter doesn't matter as long as the child learns to disregard it while focusing on the primary message
- Make sure the background noise is loud enough to be distracting but not loud enough to be painful or unpleasant.
- Decrease background competition while improving directed attention.
- To avoid fatigue and overload caused by the intense concentration required for these exercises, make sure they do not exceed fifteen minutes.

Case No. 2

Andrew was seen at the audiology clinic for a comprehensive central auditory processing assessment. Background information highlighted somewhat of an uneven developmental profile. Andrew seemed to be experiencing difficulty in expressive language skills; he was not able to formulate an appropriate response to information. This problem was accentuated by his limited vocabulary. He was unable to complete assignments and to follow directions for required tasks at school. He seemed disorganized in his work, which contributed to his inability to process information at a speed necessary to cope in the classroom. These problems were compounded by some motor coordination and balance difficulties.

At the same time, now at age eleven, Andrew was making good progress academically in such conceptual areas as math and various nonverbal problem-solving tasks. While his parents noted progress in nonverbal areas, they were still concerned about his difficulty in the expressive language domain.

Audiometric Test Results

Pure tone audiometry revealed normal hearing bilaterally. Impedance audiometry revealed normal middle ear function. Based on normal findings, a comprehensive CAP evaluation was initiated. Andrew exhibited the characteristics of an *output-organization deficit* in central auditory processing.

Output-Organization *Deficit*

This deficiency was reflected in Andrew's inability to organize, sequence, plan, and formulate appropriate responses to incoming auditory information. As far as the problem of disorganization was concerned, Andrew needed to learn how to use organizational aids, such as notebooks and calendars, as well as be exposed to strategies designed to strengthen organizational skills. Speech—language intervention services were arranged in order to address the expressive language component of his disorder.

The processes related to central auditory abilities are interdependent and interactive in that they are influenced by other stimuli, such as visual, tactile, proprioceptive, and motor. The entire brain with all of its interconnections must work in perfect synchrony for sensory integration to take place so that normal processing can occur. Though Andrew's problem could be labeled a verbal expressive language deficiency, he did show some disturbance in broader areas of intersensory integration. Therefore, a comprehensive, holistic, management approach is necessary in such a case to bring about functional change and reorganization within his central nervous system. Management should be as deficit-specific as possible, remediating those areas that are shown to be dysfunctional while at the same time building upon Andrew's auditory strengths.

Behavioral Characteristics of Children with Output-Organization *Deficit*

It is one thing to understand information but quite another to respond to it appropriately. An auditory *output-organization deficit* is a deficiency in the ability to sort, plan, and organize information to formulate an appropriate response to it. Sorting, planning, and organizing a response are neural executive function tasks, which implies that this disorder involves the frontal lobe of the brain. Children with this deficiency usually

- exhibit expressive language dysfunction which manifest itself in poor expressive skills and in difficulty formulating, ordering, or producing an appropriate response to information received.
- have difficulty with gross and fine motor planning skills such that handwriting skills may be poor.
- have difficulty in acting on incoming information when two or more elements are involved, for example, when multiple commands are expressed in a single utterance (e.g., "bring me your book and put it on my desk, then brush your teeth and go to bed after finishing your homework.")
- have difficulty starting and completing assignments due to poor organizational skills.
- have problems with multitasking, such as taking and organizing notes at the same time.
- show weakness in sound blending, sequencing, and expressive language skills, and articulation.
- have word recall or retrieval difficulties with poor sequential memory-based skills (the process by which retention of sound sequences within words and words within sentences for immediate recall is achieved.)
- are good at reading and comprehending (receptive skills), but poor at relating what was read (expressive skills).
- exhibit attention deficiency.
- find it difficult to understand speech in noisy conditions.

Management Suggestions

Intervention must be based on development of organizational skills to aid recall. Difficulty lies in the child's inability to scan memory and recall information needed for immediate use because information is poorly organized and stored in the brain.

Therapy must, therefore, focus on the following:

- Training in rules on how to organize information for easy access; imposition of external organization in class to aid in immediate recall.
- Frequent use of organizational aids such as notebooks and calendars to strengthen memory and organizational skills.

- Training in how to organize, to revisualize, or to reauditorize (say or repeat words to one's self) a task before starting it.
- Preteaching of information (it is important that information be broken down into small linguistic units when new concepts are presented in order for good organization of information to take place).
- Repetition or rephrasing but only when information is broken down into small manageable "chunks" or linguistic units for processing.
- Use of activities and aids that emphasize order or sequence to make the information easier to remember such as mnemonics, diagrams, and maps or first letters of the information, etc.
- Emphasis on verbal expression with frequent participation in language activities so that the child can develop good expressive language skills (an intensive program of language stimulation with the goal of building up sufficient extrinsic redundancy is highly recommended).
- Use of noise-tolerance techniques and training to help the child process auditory stimuli efficiently when listening in unfavorable conditions.
- Use of speech—language intervention services in order to address the expressive language component of the child's disorder.

Case No. 3

Richard was a six-year-old boy having trouble in understanding conversation in competitive listening situations. His mother indicated that he often needed to have things repeated when spoken to before he could understand what was said. He seemed confused when exposed to more that one source of information simultaneously. Richard's mother expressed concern over his poor receptive verbal language skills. His speech, writing, and reading were all affected, demonstrating an inability to interpret or to recall incoming information accurately, especially after listening for extended periods of time. She also stated that, occasionally, he would become frustrated during conversation as he seemed to forget what he wanted to say. At times, he would cover his ears to block out background noise, which seemed to severely limit his ability to focus attention on tasks at hand.

Audiometric Test Results

Cognitively, Richard had normal intelligence with no evidence of bilateral hearing loss. Speech recognition scores were 100 percent in both ears. Impedance for the assessment of middle ear function was normal bilaterally.

Observation and Conclusions

Based on normal findings of the audiometric test results, a comprehensive CAP evaluation was initiated. For most tests of central auditory processing, the older the child, the greater the chance for comparative normative data to be meaningfully interpreted. Because of Richard's age (six), interpretation of results on these tests had to be guarded. With children around six, there is a high degree of variability in results. So while it is possible to have a child tested at this age, interpretation of test results should not be as stringent as in older children.

Richard responded well to the test procedure, although at times, he became restless and unfocused, and thus the test was adjusted to achieve maximum cooperation on his part. The results were considered to be reliable and useful in pinpointing certain potential problem areas that needed to be monitored. Richard exhibited the characteristics that fit the profile of a *binaural separation and integration deficit*.

Binaural Separation and Integration Deficit

Binaural integration and separation are processes crucial to everyday listening situations, especially in a school environment, where the child must focus attention on a primary message source while ignoring or integrating competing signals in the classroom. A binaural *separation and integration deficit* manifest itself in the inability to get information from one side of the brain to the other efficiently due to poor interhemispheric connection between the right and left hemispheres of the brain.

When both hemispheres of the brain are not working synchronously, the child's ability to execute certain classroom activities simultaneously with smoothness and efficiency may be compromised. There may also be noticeable deficiencies in gross and fine motor skills. Strategies recommended, therefore, need to include not only verbal but nonverbal activities as well, with enough repetition to facilitate the efficiency of interhemispheric transfer of information via the corpus callosum.

Behavioral Characteristics of Children with Binaural Separation and Integration Deficit

Children with binaural integration and separation deficiency may display some or all of the behavioral characteristics listed below. They

- have difficulty with selective listening, get confused when more than one person is talking at a time.
- have low tolerance for background noise.

- have difficulty performing several tasks at the same time, for example, auditory—visual—motor task such as copying from the blackboard or taking dictation and holding down paper while listening to and tracking the teacher in the classroom.
- perform poorly on dichotic tasks in the central auditory processing evaluation (tasks involving the presentation of different stimuli presented simultaneously to both ears).
- at a very young age, most children process information better with the right ear than left. However, in normal listening children, the difference between ears becomes smaller as child grows older and as communication between the right and left sides of the brain becomes more efficient with maturity, while in children with binaural integration and separation deficiency that significant performance difference between ears persists.
- have poor whole-word recognition skills. They see words but cannot pronounce them without breaking them down into individual sounds.
- have difficulty extracting meaning from prosodic aspects of speech such as rhythm, intonation, and stress.
- have difficulty figuring out how to do tasks, especially tasks that require the use of more than one modality simultaneously.
- need to be shown how to do tasks repeatedly until they understand it.
- exhibit a lack of persistence and give up task easily because of difficulty.
- are unable to tolerate distraction.
- have poor motor skills (such as handwriting, where words are often improperly spaced).
- have poor musical skills.
- cannot maintain rhythmic patterns in speech and tend to jumble words.
- have poor inflectional patterns of speech (intonation), speaking in monotone (without "peaks" and "valleys.")

Management Suggestions

Management is based on helping the child with interhemispheric transfer of information across the brain. Problems that involve integration are interhemispheric by nature and management must be focused on developing efficient transfer of information across the cerebral hemispheres. Since the right hemisphere is responsible for contributing the emotional elements to speech and the left hemisphere is specialized for language, these two hemispheres must be synchronized so that the child can take advantage of the prosodic elements of speech to extract meaning.

Children with this deficiency do have difficulty understanding the subtleties of language. Studies have shown that prosodic skills can be taught (Hargrove, et al., 1989). There is a wealth of information to be derived from acoustic contours in speech, such as rhythm, stress, and intonation that cannot be determined simply from the words of a message alone. Children must learn to extract meaning from these suprasegmental elements of speech if information is to make sense to them. In the classroom, children who rely on the prosodic aspects of speech for understanding have a greater chance of processing information when presented in difficult listening conditions than those who do not. The following approaches can be helpful in stimulating this process:

- Begin with rhythm tasks on one side of the body (ex., have the child follow and maintain rhythmic patterns on a drum or similar object).
- Vary rate of beats (slow, fast, constant) imitated by the child.
- Encourage foot tapping to the rhythm of the beats.
- Progress to bilateral rhythms after the child has established rhythmic patterns on one side of the body.
- Progress to beating out rhythm with both hands and feet.
- Have the child recognize different inflectional and rhythmic patterns of speech.
- Progress to rhythm patterns of language by particular inflectional patterns being superimposed on simple phrases and sentences.
- Put stress on rhythmic patterns, including words and sentences with accent and inflectional variation.
- Train the child in the use of prosodic aspects of speech (acoustic contour), such as rhythm, stress, and intonation essential to convey meaning.
- Teach the child how to detect inflectional and rhythmic patterns of language.
- Practice on words that convey different meaning simply by using stress patterns.

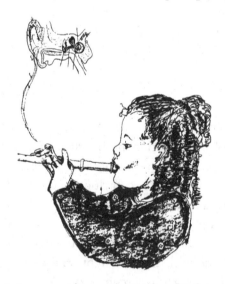

Music increases the rapid transfer of information
between the two hemispheres of the brain.

114

- Have the child attend musical instrument, singing, or dancing lessons to enhance rapid transfer of interhemispheric information between the two sides of the brain.
- When rephrasing information, add new information to the original message and repeat it with related gestures, while emphasizing stress, rhythm, and intonational patterns of the message for keyword extraction. The overall goal is to have the child comprehend social sounds, words, and meaningful verbal symbols through acoustic contours.
- Have the child identify the who, what, when, and where of the story.
- Use games requiring action in a specific pattern to improve integration and pattern recognition skills.
- Engage the child in building jigsaw puzzles or building models for conceptual purposes in order to help the child learn to relate parts to a whole.
- Pair up speech messages with music and melody to reinforce skills.
- Read poems and nursery rhymes to the child.
- Engage the child in social role playing (e.g., "What would you do if . . .")
- In the classroom, employ multisensory stimuli discretely. Environment full of visual, tactile or other stimuli may be distracting and add to confusion rather than assist in learning because of the child's inability to integrate sensory input. Too much stimulation may confuse the child rather than simplify things.
- Ensure a balance between the child's tolerance levels and the stimulation provided.
- Encourage performance of multiple tasks, such as taking notes from the blackboard while listening to information at the same time (present at speed at which the child processes).
- Regular review of learned material to strengthen neural connections between stored information in the brain.
- Try noise-tolerance techniques to help the child focus on the primary message while ignoring competing signals in the environment.

Chapter 12

Teaching Success with Children Having CAPD

Children with auditory processing difficulties often struggle in their classrooms without having their problem identified. Yet how these children are taught makes a great difference between learning and not learning. These children have normal potential and learn successfully if they are correctly taught; they simply need specialized and skilled assistance.

In general, however, teachers do not consistently identify those children in their classrooms who are learning and those who are not. Too often, it is only after exam results are reviewed that the teacher realizes that certain children have gleaned significantly little from their efforts throughout the entire school year. In one study in which teachers were asked to identify in their classes pupils with impaired hearing, they missed 15 percent of the hearing-impaired pupils while rating 5 percent of the normal hearers as hearing-impaired. In the same study, teachers failed to identify six of the most severely hearing impaired pupils sitting in their classroom daily who were failing because of a significant hearing impairment and because of inappropriate seating placement in the classroom.

The principal of the school responded to this finding by saying that if teachers were failing to correctly identify children with hearing problems in his school, then those who could surely identify them would be the parents. But a similar study found that both parents and teachers were performing slightly better than chance in identifying children with significant hearing problems. Parents and teachers were making incorrect judgments for *four* out of every *ten* children they had identified (Kodman, 1978).

What causes a child to miss significant portions of information? One theory suggests that when an acoustic waveform (sound wave) enters the ear and is changed into electrochemical impulses on its way to the brain for interpretation, some of these impulses get lost in the process (transduction loss) so that gaps are created in the sequence of impulses as they arrive at the brain, thus making it difficult for the brain to decode the incoming stimuli accurately. If this is true, it has serious implications for the child who has problems listening in noise and explains, partially at least, the difficulty they experience when listening in highly competitive environments.

This transduction loss, however, does not seem sufficient in itself to restrict the ability to process information effectively when listening conditions are degraded by noise. The reason is that the same degraded listening conditions exist with normal listening children as well, and yet these children have little difficulty processing information. However, when transduction loss is combined with external variables present in the classroom, then children with CAPD encounter enormous processing difficulties while trying to make sense of what they hear. What are those external variables in the classroom that may contribute to processing difficulties?

First, the child may have limited *memory capacity* and *perceptual speed*. Memory capacity refers to the amount of information stored per unit of time that the child can retain (store). As far as perceptual speed is concerned, every child learns differently and at a different rate. If information is presented at the child's *perceptual speed*, that is, the speed at which the child processes information, it will be assimilated (stored); if it is not, it will be lost. If the child is to adequately sequence the string of rapidly successive sounds that make up speech information, this information must be delivered within the child's perceptual speed. Only then can the brain move on to other complex tasks of storing, organizing, and retrieving the information when required to do so. When the child cannot process the sounds of language fast enough for adequate comprehension and expression to take place, he or she will be unable to develop a linguistic system effective enough for communication. When these receptive capabilities are impaired, the child will lack the tools necessary for thought, understanding, and academic achievement (More will be said on perceptual speed later in this chapter).

Second, the source from which information originates may be too distant. When distance between listener (the child) and speaker (the teacher) is too great, the intensity of the speaker's voice reaching the listener's ear is reduced, which in turn affects both clarity and localization of the teacher's voice. Too great a distance makes it difficult for the child to extract meaning from what the teacher is saying. When this practice continues on a daily basis, it has a cumulative effect on the child's ability to organize and to recall information with any degree of accuracy and precision.

Other factors that affect listening in the classroom include the following:

- The information presented may be too disorganized for the child to organize, store, and retrieve when required. The human brain scans stored information while looking for a desired response. The more organized the stored information is, the easier it will to be retrieved.
- The child may not be familiar with the material he or she is asked to process.
- Noise levels within the classroom may be influencing speech intelligibility. When noise is coupled with significant distance between the child and teacher, speech may degrade at a rate that hampers comprehension.
- The emotional and psychological state of the child may be creating internal noise build-up.

- The quality of the acoustics in the classroom may be extremely poor, and the reverberation time of speech may be too long.
- The teaching style and manner of presentation may be threatening and, therefore, may not be conducive to learning.
- The teacher's accent or speech defect may be interfering with the child's ability to comprehend.
- Problems may be compounded by the child's poor writing skills as the child struggles to keep pace with and understand the teacher while at the same time taking notes.
- The child may have to put up with continuous annoyance from peers as he or she tries to make sense of what the teacher is saying.
- The child may have an existing hearing loss, allergies, or general poor health, which means that his or her hearing may vary from day to day. Such conditions are debilitating and may contribute to the child's inattentiveness and distractibility in the classroom.

CODATION

The acronym CODATION is here to help teachers remember the very important elements needed for the teaching success of children with processing difficulties. When strategies based on these elements are implemented, marked academic strides toward achievement can be seen in the classroom:

Teaching Module	**C**larity for comprehension **O**rganization **D**elivery
Learning Module	**A**ttention **T**iming **I**ndividualized instruction **O**bservation
Environmental Modification	**N**oise—free environment (including preferential seating, good classroom acoustics for reduction of noise levels, and assistive listening devices)

Teaching module

Clarity

To fully appreciate how comprehension of auditory information takes place, one must understand how the ear works. The auditory system is constantly refining information from the time a signal (message) enters the ear canal until it reaches the brain for processing. Hearing sound is one thing, but interpreting or attributing meaning to that sound is another. Comprehension is the ability to restructure all incoming stimuli into meaningful linguistic patterns of information for understanding. But meaning is acquired only if there are no deficiencies in the input channel. A deficiency in the input channel will limit the manner in which meaning is ascribed.

The development of inner language—the language of the mind, the language with which one thinks—depends on normal receptive processes. Without this inner language, children cannot ascribe substance, meaning, or significance to what they hear and speak. This is developed in the process of communication where input precedes output. In other words, comprehension or receptive language precedes expressive language in the normal developmental process of communication. Any interruption of the input and output interchange seriously influences children's ability to effectively communicate the information received. When problems are present, focus must, therefore, be placed primarily on improving the child's decoding ability as well as his or her encoding skills for the effective management of information. To this end, information must be properly processed so that it can be recalled and be given back accurately. Teachers can aid in this process in two important ways.

First, teachers should maximize audibility (the clarity of information reaching the child's ear). This is achieved through improving the effectiveness of the delivery system in the classroom. The information must first be clear to the children if they are to express themselves accurately. In other words, what goes in (input) must be clearly understood in order for it to be correctly and accurately expressed (output).

The ability to adequately express one's self is crucially linked to the ability to understand the spoken word. When comprehension is attained through correct analysis and proper integration of information, verbal expression naturally follows as a logical consequence. This input and output interchange is necessary for the proper developmental progression from listening to effective speech and then on to reading and finally to writing, all of which depend on the normal development of inner language.

Second, teachers should ensure that comprehension has been achieved by frequently testing for understanding. By requiring children to reproduce what they have heard, teachers can see not only whether the information has been properly conceptualized but also whether it can be accurately reproduced through expression. Children who cannot express themselves adequately have a verbal expressive deficiency. They are limited in their ability to organize, sequence, recall, and later express information they received with accuracy.

Teachers must therefore ensure that both reception and expression are unaffected at the time of information delivery. A simple test of understanding involves repeating information or rephrasing it when children show lapses in comprehension and then requiring them to paraphrase what they heard. Teachers must always be aware that children with auditory perceptual or listening disorders often have some delay in language development. The questioning and paraphrasing is an important activity by the teacher because it ensures that comprehension has taken place and that the information has been assimilated sufficiently to be appropriately expressed.

Organization

Recall of information is achieved through the neural process of scanning. *Scanning* is the ability to survey the storage of auditory experiences and match previous data with the present auditory experience. When neural impulses reach the brain for processing, they arrive with signatures (codes) that the brain directs to Heschl's gyrus, the vast auditory reception region of the auditory cortex. This auditory reception region is a huge signal processor with interconnected neural pathways extending to various centers within the cerebral cortex.

In order to readily establish a match with previous concepts, information is rapidly compared with a set of similar features that are stored in long-term memory through the process of scanning. But previous information must be properly stored in order to be effectively retrieved. If a comparison cannot be found immediately, the brain initiates a second state of comparisons in quick succession, focusing on the defining features of the incoming information. When an adequate overlap of these features is attained, comparison is achieved (Rips, et. al., 1973; Smith, et. al., 1974). This is an extremely vital central auditory processing function related to memory and to learning.

Therefore, the more organized the material when it is presented by the teacher, the more efficiently the brain can store the information, and the easier it is for it to be retrieved when looking for a desired response through scanning. Perceptual learning is best facilitated by presenting information systematically and requiring immediate feedback. All material presented to children with CAPD should, therefore, be conveyed in a well-organized and systematic manner in order to improve both comprehension and auditory memory. Thus teachers must make sure that the input material is presented not only clearly but also in a sequentially organized manner to enhance the brain's ability to scan its store of information and efficiently retrieve it when needed.

Delivery

Every child learns differently and at a different rate because each individual's brain is wired differently for learning. Therefore, the information delivery system of the teacher must be constantly monitored to ensure that it matches the child's processing capabilities. The question of *how* information is being communicated to the child at any given time must not be taken lightly. The speed of visual and auditory processing, known as *perceptual speed*, plays an important role in the child's ability to conceptualize that information. If the central auditory nervous system is to integrate incoming information efficiently and store it for future recall, the way the information is presented must match the speed of the child's processing capabilities. Therefore, before teaching takes place the following questions should be answered.

- What is this child's information handling capacity?
- Is there too much information at a time, exceeding the child's capacity to store it?
- Is the information being presented so rapidly that it does not match up with the child's processing capabilities?
- If so, at what speed can it be more effectively transmitted?

When information is presented in a well-paced, well-articulated, and organized manner, child processes it and retains it. Teachers are the facilitators of this process. By using simple, well-constructed sentences delivered in manageable "chunks" tailored to the child's level of comprehension and perceptual speed, they allow them to comprehend and store information for future use. *Chunking*—the breaking down and organizing information into small, manageable bits for easy assimilation—is highly recommended. This approach makes it possible for information to be conceptualized because information is delivered at the rate at which the child process it and retains it.

Presenting too much information too rapidly when children are capable of retaining only small amounts at a time results in confusion, information loss, and a general breakdown in attention to events of importance. It causes the children's mind to shift fleetingly and randomly from one internal event to another without focus. Eventually, children simply stop listening or processing altogether. Their attention wander in the classroom, and they become detached and distracted by ambient stimuli, which makes it difficulty to follow instructions for completing tasks. Often these children are described as daydreamers and are said to be absent-minded, since they cannot remember what they have been told. Valuable instruction time is lost under these circumstances.

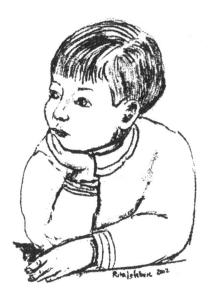

With too much information the child may stop listening or processing altogether.

It is important to remember that children with central auditory processing disorders process information at a much slower rate than those with normal processing capabilities. Therefore, it is imperative that the delivery system of information be matched with their specific processing speed.

For this reason, teachers should experiment with their delivery system by varying the speed of presentation and the amount of information presented at a time. By so doing, they can determine the rate at which information should be delivered to a particular child. They can then deliver information to match the child's perceptual speed. This adjustment is extremely important if the child is to grasp, retain, and subsequently retrieve information intelligently. In the average classroom environment, where a certain amount of confusion exists and where there is a persistent flow of information, it is important for teachers to take note of the rate at which information is delivered and also the rate at which each child processes that information.

Style of presentation

Since each child learns differently, teachers must adjust their approaches to accommodate the child's strengths and weaknesses. Some children are visual learners, others are auditory learners, while others are tactile (hands-on) learners. Teachers must identify how each child learns and facilitate the process of learning by exploiting the child's strengths.

Teachers must always be cautious of where they stand when presenting information. For example, when presenting information to a visual or auditory learner, they must not stand talking with their face to the blackboard or walking around the room while the child is trying to take notes. Moreover, they should never stand where the light source is affecting the child's line of vision. The rapidity and invisibility of certain lip movements, poor lighting conditions, and distance between speaker and listener present real problems for the children who must depend on both auditory and visual cues for perception. Perception only partly dependants on the auditory system; much of it also relies on the keenness of visual acuity to supplement auditory cues.

To improve understanding, visual and auditory cues should be used in such a way that they supplement each other for improved understanding. The importance of visual cues cannot be overstressed. Visual cues can greatly help when the teacher's voice is enmeshed in classroom noise and when speech intelligibility is a problem. The ability to see the teacher when listening in noise contributes significantly to children's perception of what the teacher is saying. Therefore teachers must always be assured that they have the visual and auditory attention of pupils before imparting information. When listening is a challenge, other stimuli such as situational, contextual, and linguistic cues can also be used for enhanced understanding. They all play a vital role in perception especially when decoding skills are compromised.

Finally, the signal-to-noise ratio—the relationship between the intensity of a signal (teacher's voice) and noise present—must always be considered. As distance between the teacher and the child increases, the intensity of a signal is reduced. When the teacher is busy attending to the needs of other pupils in a large classroom area, every time they walk away from the student with a listening problem, the intensity of her message is reduced, and a reduced signal induces signal delay, which in turn increases distortion of that signal as it reaches the brain.

Attention

Children with an attention deficit generally fail to focus on a certain amount of information that is heard or read. Children who fail to focus for prolonged periods of time are said to have a short attention span. They cannot retain more than a certain amount of information in proper sequence for purposes of immediate action or recall. Children with a limited memory span disorder, generally fail to execute commands or instructions because they cannot retain a series of instructions long enough to execute them. This in turn affects how they understand things. Certain issues concerning such children must be addressed before any teaching takes place. The following questions should be answered:

- How long can this child listen before he loses attention altogether?
- Are the elements in the environment—auditory or visual or both—that can be distracting?
- What stimuli help the child focus and maintain attention?

- When he relies on auditory alone, how well does he or she process information?
- When auditory and visual stimuli are combined, is the child's performance improved or impeded?
- How well does the child retain a series of instructions?
- Is the child capable of executing a series of commands?

The control of attention is a primary objective for teachers. The main problem in this regard is that often children do not recognize when they have stopped listening and quickly forget what they have heard. Teachers must fight against this tendency. When attention can be achieved over time, it eventually reprograms a brain that is unfocused and not used to being selective in what it processes.

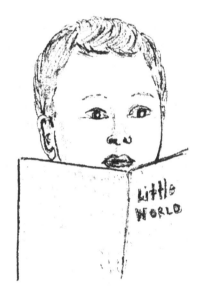

The teacher must always be alert for attention lapses.

The presence of distractions along with all other competing elements operating in the learning environment must be minimized since they compete for children's attention. Distraction diminishes concentration level and diverts the children's attention away from the primary source of information, which is the teacher's voice. In order to maximize attention, teachers must constantly be aware of what distracters are present in the listening and learning environment and how they affect the children's ability to focus. If they do not aid learning, these distractions must be removed from the learning area.

Helping children achieve selective focus of attention is always a challenge and requires great skill. The process is facilitated by gaining children's attention before presenting material. Teachers devise various strategies for achieving this goal. For example, before presenting information, a teacher may tap a pencil to indicate that he or she is ready to present new material and requires undivided attention. When changing topics, a teacher may give verbal or physical cues, which stimulate the RAS and prepare it for the reception of incoming information. It is important to help children understand the importance of these commands.

During instruction, teachers should always be on the alert for signs of fatigue and lack of concentration by spotting attention lapses in their pupils. Children with listening disorders have great difficulty maintaining focus while extracting information from background noise, especially when they have been engaged over prolonged periods of time.

Another way of securing optimum attention is by improving speech intelligibility in the classroom. Teachers can adjust the intensity of their voice to the amount of background noise present in the classroom by reducing the distance between themselves and the children, while increasing the distance between children and their distracting peers. All noise in the listening area must be reduced or controlled. This enhances the signal-to-noise ratio, leading to improved speech intelligibility.

When children do not process information in the classroom as a result of inattention, this results not only in significant delays in their mental development, but it causes a generalized breakdown in all (encoding) aspects of perception. These children will persistently lag behind their peers in performance as information is lost and as valuable time is wasted while they try to catch up with others in the class.

Adding to the child's failure to comprehend, may be his poor handwriting skills which causes him to further lag behind as the teacher dispenses information he struggles to write. The inability to direct full attention to the spoken word and record information simultaneously virtually ensures that these children will miss a great portion of what the teacher says. The problem with taking class notes is in fact twofold. First, children cannot remember what they have heard since they cannot retain a series of instructions long enough to get it down on paper. Second, because of their forgetfulness, they fail to comprehend the information coming from the teacher, which they receive only in fragments. Therefore, by the time the teacher is finished, there are too many gaps in the information to make sense of what was said.

These gaps in information inevitably cause children to stop trying as they become easily lost in the classroom. Thus they continue to fall behind their peers who have long processed the information and have gone on to other instructions presented before they had time to catch up. This forces them to ask to have things repeated and explained over and over again much to the exasperation of the teacher, who often finds such behavior disruptive and time-consuming.

Teachers can devise certain strategies to minimize these difficulties. For example, they can have a child use the notes of another note-taker in the classroom who is more adept at this task. Children who have difficulty with taking notes should be encouraged to do this so that they can supplement their own notes with those of the other child. (It is important, however, that the teacher review those notes for accuracy when the class session is over.) This arrangement is referred to as the "buddy system." It can be very effective in many ways in assisting children who have difficulty keeping pace with the rest of the class.

Another suggestion for dealing with the problem of delayed performance due to inattention is to have the teacher preteach the new topic before presenting it for formal discussion to the class. This strategy helps increase familiarity with the subject beforehand. Children can also be provided with the lecture notes prior to the class presentation so that they can become familiar with the new concepts pertaining to the discussion before they are introduced in the classroom. When children are familiar with the topic of discussion before hand, their understanding of it when it is presented greatly increases. They are better able to decode certain words or even phonemes of a sentence as a result of prior rehearsal. Prior knowledge of the subject, therefore, facilitates the total perception of the subject, making the information easier to understand when it is presented, even under the most difficult listening conditions.

Since children with CAPD do not have the same facility with language as normal children do, they often have a difficult time understanding concepts when presented for the first time, especially if the listening environment is compromised. Thus, with all new topics, a brief discussion of the new information beforehand is always helpful. A summary immediately after the discussion also helps, allowing the teacher to aid the learning process by highlighting important points on the chalkboard to reinforce what has been taught.

Furthermore, to increase participation in the classroom, teachers can familiarize these children with new vocabulary and select keywords from the discussion to be used during the spelling lesson or in sentences during other classes. These strategies help the children determine by context which words are being used when the new topic is under discussion, especially when listening is difficult. This is sure to increase participation on the part of children and minimize inattention even though listening conditions may be less than ideal at the time when the new topic is being taught.

Timing

The process of developing new concepts with children at the appropriate time is very important. The thing to remember is that concept formation (thinking and reasoning) is developed slowly. Concept formation is a process that children gradually acquire as they begin to comprehend, analyze, and generalize information from one learning situation to the next. To facilitate this process, teachers must review past material before presenting new material so that the children establish relationships and associations (linkage) between previous and present learning.

Regular and systematic review of material allows children to form lasting relationships between information past and information present. Such links increase their ability to process rapidly and efficiently. Reviewing information is a sure way of reinforcing concepts already learned. It makes it much easier for children to grasp and retain new information even when listening conditions are not conducive to learning. When listening in noise, children who reviewed information they have learned can more easily recognize certain words and concepts mentioned by relying on context to make sense of what they are hearing. In short, as a result of reviewing, previous concepts become more meaningful and are more permanently established.

Nothing is more vital in strengthening weak neural connections between information in the brain than the teacher's use of a developmental sequential strategy, reinforced by a thorough review of past information before the presentation of new material. Such an approach not only strengthens neural connection in the brain but also develops neurological processes for the organization and retention of new ideas. When information is reviewed, the ability to generalize information and engage in conceptual thinking is greatly accelerated.

Finally, the experiential learning approach is best suited to these children's needs for acquiring new ideas and concepts. Since children with CAPD have difficulty attributing meaning and significance to sound, they inevitably have difficulty acquiring and using language. It is helpful to teach them how to associate sound with the proper units of experience. For example, from very early in the child's development, expose the child to everyday sounds in their environment and associate them with some relevant experience. For example, take the child to the window as a plane flies over. Familiarize him or her with the sounds of the home, school, and zoo. Have him use the blender at home, pencil sharpener, and other instruments until he eventually relates objects to experiences. This approach requires a coordinated effort between home and school with both caregivers and teachers working together to provide the child with a rich learning experience gleaned form everyday life situations outside and within the confines of the classroom.

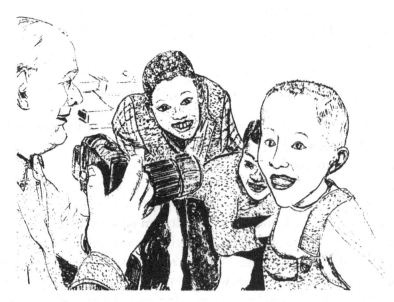

The experimental approach to learning is best in acquiring new ideas and concepts.

Individualized Instruction

Individualized instruction is one of the most effective ways of improving children's focus and productivity. Individual sessions are the ideal time for the child to develop the power of concentration and focused attention-powers that are stymied in the noisy classroom environment. When a child is studying alone with the instructor and knows that he or she will be required to recall information, the child's listening habits are generally improved.

However, it must be stressed here that while this is an important strategy for teaching children who may be experiencing difficulty with concentration in the noisy classrooms, it is desirable for these children to associate with others with normal processing capabilities as much as possible. It is from these children that a child with concentration and listening problems gets assistance in certain schoolwork activities, especially the language arts, and in many ways, learn to model the way the normal listening child manages incoming information.

One advantage of individualized instruction is that the teacher can repeat information that the child might have missed in the classroom environment. Children with perceptual listening problems always seem to perform better on one-on-one basis with their tutor, than in the large, noisy environments such as the classroom setting. It is best to use this opportunity, therefore, to introduce new subject matter with significant thought content.

Periodic checks of the child's understanding should be made, even under the quiet listening conditions of one-on-one sessions, to ensure that the information has been properly assimilated. Teachers should encourage children to repeat instructions to themselves as they work alone. This is especially important when reading is involved. Subvocalization (reauditorization) in reading should be encouraged until the child's reading skills have improved sufficiently to eliminate this practice. When subvocalization is used, the basic sounds of language are constantly heard and mentally reinforced by the child through the auditory channel. The technique can also be applied to spelling: the child should say the word while writing it. Another advantage of subvocalization is that it helps the teacher, speech pathologist, or whoever is in charge of the management of the child to analyze the types or errors the child makes (ex., substitutions and omissions) as well as monitor problems with phrasing, punctuation, and meaning.

Not all children can benefit from subvocalization, however, so the decision to use this strategy should always be weighed carefully and made on an individual basis. There are those who can read silently but not orally; others must read aloud to comprehend. Each child must be evaluated to determine his or her particular strengths and needs and the most effective means of dealing with the problem.

Individualized instruction is an ideal time to fill in gaps in language and other areas of deficiency stemming from the child's inability to do so within the large noisy classroom setting. When the teacher perceives that the child has not processed certain information in the group session, individualized instruction is the most effective way to cover that material.

Individualized instruction requires a great deal of cooperation between the classroom teacher and the child's special teacher or tutor so that they can coordinate instructional plans for the child. Children with CAPD who receive individualized instruction are far more focused and productive in their performance.

Observation

As has been mentioned earlier, teachers of children with listening disorders must constantly watch for signs of fatigue and lack of concentration, attention, and comprehension. Teachers cannot expect absolute attention at all times, however, because listening is hard work. Even children without processing difficulties tire and fatigue when listening in strenuous conditions.

Furthermore, some children hear better on some days than on others due to the child's mental, physical, and emotional state at the time. Teacher must be careful not to misinterpret children's inattention as lack of interest and motivation as has been alluded to earlier. To prevent fatigue and inattentiveness, the teacher should permit frequent pauses during lesson sessions so that children can relax and recover.

Children with impaired auditory function tire quickly from listening because of the effort it takes to compete and keep pace with their peers while engaged in classroom activities. Both vision and auditory senses are taxed to the maximum trying to cope with information presented in highly competitive conditions.

When children with auditory processing difficulties are tired, they naturally process poorly because of the high level of stress and anxiety they experience as they try to keep up with others while at the same time concentrating on everything the teacher is saying. Prolong periods of concentration cause them to attend sporadically to information with noticeable lapses. During instruction, therefore, teachers should constantly monitor these children's attention level. As mentioned above, they should provide short, intensive periods of instruction and allow break intervals during which children can move around freely to recover from the stress of listening. Above all, the children's progress should be evaluated on a regular and systematic basis so that the program in which they are engaged can be modified and adjusted whenever necessary to meet each child's particular needs.

Environmental Modifications

Noise-free environment

Even within the environment of the school, it has become increasingly difficult to find a place of quiet retreat for reflection and creative thought. Those quiet periods that give the over stimulated hair cells of the inner ear a chance to recover from the impact of excessive noise pollution throughout the day are hard to find within the confines of the school. And noise, regardless of its intensity, has an effect on academic performance.

Whenever noise interferes with communication, it must be considered when measuring a child's performance and productivity in the classroom. Its effect on performance in the classroom is insidious and cumulative but as dangerous as any other health hazard found in our air or water today. Yet its dangers have been minimized, neglected, and not communicated effectively to date. Thus it has been tolerated and its consequences in the classroom have remained illusive and largely ignored over the years, though its effects can be lasting and devastating.

Annoyance caused by noise is usually greater indoors than outdoors, and it usually increases as the level and frequency of the noise increase. That is why noise is such a significant factor within the confines of the classroom. Noise affects both memory and capacity to learn and its impact is greater when speech is involved. The reason for this is that noise acts as a masker in the classroom, raising the threshold for speech intelligibility. In other words, the listener (the child) often behaves as a hearing-impaired person requiring louder speech above the noise levels in order to understand what is being said.

If intense enough, background noise can make the speech signal unintelligible or, in some instances, confuse the listener by altering the direction from which the speech is originating. What is worse, it can obliterate the speech signal altogether. The primary questions teachers should ponder, therefore, as far as classroom acoustics are concerned are the following:

- To what extent does background noise affect the child's ability to process?
- Does the child have the ability to suppress irrelevant information while focusing on relevant stimuli?
- How well can the child attend selectively to a particular stimulus embedded within other stimuli originating from two or more different sources at once?
- Can the child readily localize sound and easily identify the source of speech sounds in the noisy environment?

This last question deals with the concept of *sound localization* and its relevance to speech in noise. Since localization of sound has important implications for performance in situations where the teacher's voice is enmeshed in background noise, it warrants further discussion here. The localization of sound, preferential seating, classroom acoustics, and assistive listening devices which are examined later, are all influenced by the child's ability to determine the direction from which sound originates.

Localization of Sound

Localization ability is a vital function of speech perception and is indispensable in the process of attending to speech in noise. It is a very important function for children trying to distinguish and interpret speech signals in competitive listening situations, where the teacher's voice must constantly be identified. In order to interpret sound, children must first be able to localize it. They must first know where exactly the speech signals are originating.

Many children have great difficulty understanding information in noise because of impaired auditory localization function. In other words, they have difficulty locating the source of direction of sound in noisy listening environments. This is particularly the case in group conversations where there may be more than one speaker at a time. Therefore, it is important to know how localization works in order to understand the role it plays in these children's auditory perception.

There are several key factors that contribute to localization. For one, the listener must have two normally functioning ears. If one ear is functional, and the other is not, the individual has difficulty identifying the sound source. Moreover, the spatial separation of ears on the head, provides assistance in identifying the same sound somewhat differently between the ears; this constitute an important element in sound localization function. Furthermore, localization is possible because sound waves travel much slower than light waves, so there is some difference between the sound arriving at one ear compared to the other ear. Another contributing factor is that a sound containing high frequencies is louder at the ear nearer to it, than it is at the farther ear. The difference becomes less as the sound source approaches the center of the head, where both ears hear the same sound equally. When this occurs, we can always tell when a sound is directly in front or somewhere behind us even with our eyes closed.

All of these conditions are operative only because of normally functioning ears. Under these conditions, an individual can integrate acoustic information from both ears for speech when he knows where the speech is origination and can better orient himself to process it. In unilateral hearing, where one ear is normal and the other is not, both ears are out of synchrony with each other, which creates serious localization problems for the listener.

The auditory nerve in the low brainstem have the greatest impact on localization function. Children with certain listening disorders such as CAPD are unable to process the information they receive, due to impaired localization function at the brainstem level. Their inability to localize speech impairs their judgment in detecting speech in noise and makes it very difficult for them to suppress stimuli that are not relevant to the message. This inability to suppress irrelevant stimuli may be responsible for their deficiencies in figure-ground discrimination tasks, making them unable to extract meaning from signals that are enmeshed in noise. Noise tolerance training mentioned earlier may be helpful here for children learning to suppress irrelevant stimuli in the noisy classroom setting.

Preferential Seating

Preferential seating in the classroom can be defined as a placement that puts the child in a position that best accommodates his or her particular auditory needs and that best facilitates learning in the least restrictive manner. Because it optimizes the seating arrangement for easy access to information, preferential seating is an effective means of enhancing children's listening capabilities. Only when children are always in a position where they can constantly track both their teacher and their classmates, can they expend only minimum effort in trying to achieve understanding. But even when preferential seating is used, noise levels must be constantly monitored and controlled, particularly when activities require much thought and intense concentration.

When determining the options for classroom placement for the child, the management team should considered the following factors:

- The acoustics of the classroom relative to noise levels.
- Reverberation and the teacher's communication style.
- The type of structure used in the classroom: In general, a self-contained, structured classroom is more effective for children with auditory processing difficulties, than an open, unstructured teaching environment.
- The exact position that will maximize visual and auditory cues so that the child is constantly able to monitor both teacher and classmates with relative ease while receiving a clear, high fidelity, speech signal.

Hence, placement of the child must be based on needs that are periodically and objectively assessed, and not on the basis of administrative convenience. Parents must insist that there child is not confined to an inappropriate setting simply because appropriate administrative alternatives have not been created by an administration that considers such alternatives too expensive.

As the child's needs change so should his placement. What is needed is a transformation form an environment of failure to one that generates success. It must become an interactive and explorative environment where teacher and student discover new things about themselves and the world, and where new ideas are generated and realistic goals are set and met from both teacher and child alike. This necessitates a broad and interesting curriculum, a balanced program of extracurricular activities and above all a large measure of faith in the child's ability to succeed.

Classroom Acoustics

Classroom space should be designed to

- minimize distraction
- reduce noise levels
- and provide a favorable signal-to-noise ratio for children functioning within the space

The goal here is to maintain speech levels sufficiently above hearing thresholds, while at the same time reducing ambient noise levels to the point where information can be transmitted to the students with maximum intelligibility. Actually, teaching under such conditions is beneficial to all students in the classroom, not just those who have auditory processing difficulties.

Figure 11.1

Signal-to-noise levels: The relationship between the intensity of signal and noise from the most favorable (condition 1) to least favorable (condition 3)

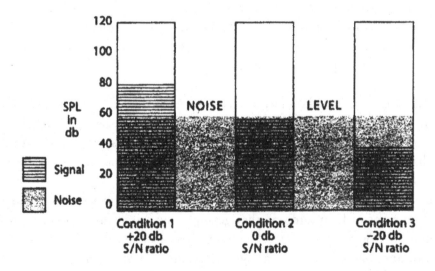

Let us consider briefly the three primary factors that generally affect speech intelligibility in the classroom. There are

- excessive noise levels
- reverberation-time within the room
- shape of the classroom space

The level of noise can be minimized by using simple techniques. Loudness can generally be controlled by alterations in the shape and size of the room and by the manner in which the room is acoustically treated. Most classrooms are relatively small, rectangular in shape, untreated, and noisy. The noise is usually augmented by hard walls, untreated floors, and flat ceilings which cause reverberation. Under these conditions, noise is reflected back and forth before reaching the ear, which makes students feel that the noise is coming from all directions.

Reverberation should be addressed first. To control reverberation, classrooms can be treated with sound absorbing materials that reduce sound reflection so that sound moves directly from its source to the listener's ear. Carpeted floors inhibit the generation of air-borne and structure-borne noise from chairs and feet, absorbing the noise and preventing it from reaching the ear. Drapes, padded seats, and acoustically treated ceiling tiles that may extent down to the height of the chair rail all help to reduce noise levels. A hard surface on the wall in the form of a chalkboard is advisable, particularly in long rooms since it helps to project the teacher's voice to the rear of the room when the teacher is talking at the blackboard. Rectangular-shaped rooms with flat or convex surfaces provide the best acoustical conditions.

A lot of window space also assists in reducing noise levels as well as allowing for better lighting in the study area. Windows and doors should be spaced as far as possible from those of adjacent classrooms to avoid spillover of noise. They should be closed during classroom sessions to avoid interclassroom interference. If they must be opened during classroom activity, they should not lead to areas where noise levels are excessive.

Ideally, the classroom space should be designed in such a way that allows a constant signal such as the teacher's voice to be sustained above the level of noise that may be present. The teacher's voice should be a clear and undistorted signal at all times and be above the level of noise that may be present. There is a word of caution here, however, one must avoid providing so much acoustic treatment that speech cannot be effectively projected in the room as this defeats the purpose for which acoustic treatment was intended in the first place.

To allow good reception, ambient noise levels should not exceed 30-35 dBA, which is equivalent to soft conversational speech with the classroom empty and with normal activity in adjacent areas. Most classrooms, however, are afflicted with environmental noise levels well surpassing this criteria. Some classrooms make it virtually impossible for children to listen and indeed learn because of intolerable noise levels.

Assistive Listening Devices

Finally, in group sessions or in large, noisy areas, assistive listening devices may be helpful in improving the listening and attention levels of children with listening disorders. When they are used, the teacher does not have to raise her voice to get the child's attention since they mildly amplify and enhance the teacher's voice above the level of background noise.

The personal FM system delivers a cleaner, clearer signal for processing by pulling the signal away from the noise; in other words, it enhances the signal and pushes the noise into the listener's perceptual background. This improves the signal-to-noise ratio for speech intelligibility, which in turn aids auditory attention and memory. Personal FM devices can be extremely effective when used strategically.

Above all, because good social relations and the attainment of social maturity are vital for children with CAPD, it is important to encourage these children to participate in school activities and social functions whenever possible in order to engender personal growth and social interaction. There is no substitute for friendships and associations formed with other children, which foster feelings of belonging and equality. Such interpersonal relationships helps to develop children's sense of self-perception, person perception, and social perception in that they allow children not only to come to terms with their own feelings but also recognize and identify with the attitudes and feelings of others. If they cannot achieve this, their emotional disturbance may become a more serious problem than that of academic underachievement.

Epilogue

One can sum by up saying that children's use and development of listening and language skills are driven by their need to communicate from the time they enter the world. The early years of life is preoccupied with sound and with attributing meaning to it. They are indeed *Listening Children*. However, disorders of the central auditory nervous system can occur from a wide range of causes, all of which are not yet precisely understood.

Some of these behaviors may result from severe forms of pathology due to specific central lesions of the brain, while others may simply be related to abnormal auditory behaviors due to lack of proper environmental stimulation. Whatever the cause, children's intellectual development may be restricted causing them to function at a suboptimal level impeding their ability to think and to learn normally with important implications for reading and language development.

It was once assumed that children learned normally as long as they had functional sight and hearing and as long as their mental capacities were in tact. Then came central auditory processing disorders around the 1950s and 1960s. It was noted that certain children seem to have a performance deficiencies in information processing of auditory signals to the brain not attributed to hearing or visual impairment. These children generally had difficulty making sense of what they heard so that auditory functioning both verbally and non-verbally on an expressive, receptive or (integrative) inner language level was affected. Thus the term *central auditory processing disorder.*

A CAP disorder is not ADHD, or dyslexia, but exists as a separate entity with its own idiosyncratic characteristics. But although the child responds inconsistently to sound and may be inattentive, he or she must be distinguished from the deaf, autistic, or the child with ADHD. Children experiencing CAPD reflect an impaired ability to attend, to discriminate, to recognize, and to remember information presented auditorily even though they are of normal intelligence with unimpaired hearing function.

The child's primary difficulty is that of learning through an inefficiently transmitting auditory channel. Something intercepts information between the ear and the brain, thus rendering the child incapable of properly translating sound into language. It is believed that the neural circuits supporting language are poorly connected and are incapable of rooting incoming signals to the proper designation for processing. The result is poor speech discrimination and improper storage and retrieval capability. This limits the child from making proper use of what he hears for academic purposes and produces a generalized effect on functional behavior *in the following areas:*

- disturbance in perception
- disturbance in concept formation (thinking and reasoning)
- disturbance in language
- disturbance in emotional behavior (Johnson and Myklebust, 1971)

This condition has the effect of reducing children's total learning experience and place limits on their social maturity and social relationships as they unsuccessfully strive to win acceptance by adults and peers. Left unattended, they never seem to reach full maturity, lacking the tools for adjustment and understanding.

Audiologist are keenly interested in the perceptual abilities of children with CAPD. Their primary concerns are the following:

- Is this child's auditory channel working efficiently?
- Can the auditory channel be relied upon for the efficient transmission of information to the brain?
- Do the auditory tests administered show that the child can retain the sequence in a series of auditory stimuli and can recall and repeat them with accuracy?
- Can generalizations be inferred from the special auditory tests concerning classroom performance?
- Can this child localize environmental sounds and can he or she readily localize the source of speech sounds in his or her environment?
- What is the maturational level of the child's central auditory system and central auditory abilities at this time?

All of these issues are vital when considering the development of listening and learning in today's competitive educational environment. The purpose of central auditory assessment is to address the above concerns. It attempts to isolate the presence of a processing disorder and describe it. Once this is done, a specific management program can and must be implemented that is tailor-fitted to meet the child's specific auditory needs. Management is aimed at meeting the unusual demands of these children without labeling them as unintelligent or emotionally disturbed. How they learn to a large extent depend on how they are taught. They learn successfully if taught correctly. Neurologically, their brain is programmed for learning. The primary therapeutic goal is to achieve an auditory language system that can help them understand what they hear.

Finally, let me emphasize that a child experiencing <u>perceptual</u> disorders is endowed with a brain like any other child—a brain that is marvelously and intricately designed with a remarkable capacity for coping with massive abundance of information. In the child who is perceptually impaired something has intercepted information to the brain's processing centers and in so doing has diminished the child's ability to perform with the efficiency of his or her peers in similar listening conditions. These obstacles need to be identified, isolated, and removed. When they are, the child will listen and learn with amazing facility. But when they are not removed the child's poor self-esteem and his subaverage academic performance are intricately interrelated and form an integral part of his overall developmental delay. Management must be focused on rebuilding self-confidence from an image that has been shattered by a revolving cycle of failure!

Glossary

Afferent pathway sensory nerve fiber transmission to the brain.

Agraphia the inability to write.

Alexia the inability of the musculature for speech production to produce phonemes or for individuals to read or even comprehend the spoken word.

Ambient noise the ever-present noise of the environment.

Assistive listening devices (ALD) personal and sound field FM systems used to mildly amply the speaker's voice above the level of background noise for improved listening by the child in the classroom.

Audibility the clarity of information reaching the ear.

Audition the basic avenue through which an individual maintains contact with his environment through sound.

Auditory associative deficiency the inability to understand and successfully manipulate the complexity of language.

Auditory attention deficiency an inability to focus purposefully on incoming information for an extended period of time.

Auditory closure the ability of the child with normal auditory processing skills to achieve meaning immediately, without analysis, even though there are gaps in the message heard.

Auditory confusion this is a breakdown in the organizational and selective processes of the system so that the child is incapable of structuring the mass of incoming impulse.

Auditory decoding deficiency the inability of the brain to perceive (configure) as a whole a message even though parts are omitted or distorted by interference.

Auditory memory the ability to retain and recall the sequence of sounds within words and words within sentences upon retrieval when needed. This is critical for language development, comprehension, and expression.

Auditory memory disorder the inability to retain an amount of information in proper sequence for the purpose of immediate recall.

Auditory perception the moment-to-moment process by which incoming impulses are organized into meaningful bits of information in the brain, which are then combined with data from other sensory modalities and past experiences, to help an individual maintain awareness of his surroundings.

Auditory reception region the primary auditory reception area that receives auditory signals for processing of information.

Auditory retention deficiency failure to retain a certain amount of information heard or read.

Babbling a continuous free experimenting with speech sound that the infant engages in before the formal development of speech and language.

Basilar membrane that part of the inner ear that plays an important role in pitch perception.

Central auditory abilities those processes that take place beyond the level of hearing that are required for sound to take on meaning.

Central auditory perceptual disorder (CAPD) a deficiency in signal reception that diminishes the capacity of the central auditory nervous system to identify, select, separate, integrate, clarify, store, and retrieve, information appropriately even though there is normal hearing.

Comprehension the ability to make sense of what is heard.

Concept formation a latticeworkwork of interrelationships formed as a result of combined data from sensory modalities and past experiences.

Conductive hearing loss any disorder limited to the outer and middle ear which interferes with the transmission of sound energy through the middle to create a hearing loss.

Decoding the process of extracting meaning from auditory stimuli received by the ear.

Dichotic listening two different messages presented to both ears simultaneously.

Direct signal a signal arriving at the ear of the listener directly from its source.

Encoding the process by which ideas are translated into words.

Expressive language ability to formulate a response through the spoken word.

Figure-ground discrimination the ability to attend selectively to a particular stimulus when it is embedded within another stimuli originating from two or more different sources, and the ability to shift attention between two sources of auditory stimuli, the primary stimulus being the figure, with the secondary stimulus becoming the ground.

Functional behavior a thorough knowledge of the whole child's behavior, including his idiosyncrasies, defects, interests, and emotions.

Hearing an activity of the auditory system that receives sound as stimuli to be processed and interpreted by the auditory centers of the brain.

Hearing threshold the point at which a stimulus is just sufficient to be perceived or to produce a response.

Indirect signal a signal arriving at the ear of the listener indirectly after reflecting off surrounding surfaces—*see reverberation*.

Information overload a situation that occurs when the senses deliver more information than the central nervous system can handle (integrate); information received through one system impedes integration of that received through another.

Inner language the ability to ascribe meaning or symbolic significance to incoming information dependent on adequate receptive processes for its development.

Integration and separation deficiency inability of the left and right hemispheres of the brain along with other sensory centers of the brain to communicate.

Internal noise any internal condition—physical, emotional, or mental—that interferes with the normal reception of sound to the ear.

Listening the process by which auditory stimuli are interpreted in a meaningful and discriminative manner at the cortex.

Localization the ear's ability to locate a sound source in its immediate sound field.

Memory the ability to retain and recall that which has been learned, and may be divided into both short-term and long-term processes.

Mixed hearing loss part conductive and part sensorineural hearing loss.

Noise superfluous, unwanted, or random sound energy of various intensities and frequencies of a waveform.

Organization-output deficiency a deficiency in the ability to sequence, to plan, and to organize information for an appropriate response.

Perceptual speed the rate at which auditory cues are processed per unit of time.

Phoneme the smallest unit of speech sounds in language that distinguishes one utterance from another that affects meaning.

Phonemic awareness the ability to detect, to compare, and to manipulate phonemes in syllables and in words.

Plasticity (CNS) the nervous system's ability to undergo organizational change in response to internal and external change.

Preferential seating a seating arrangement in the classroom facilitates learning without restriction.

Prelinguistic before the acquisition of language.

Prosody the suprasegmental elements of speech such as pitch, loudness, rhythm, intonation, and stress.

Reauditorization ability to retrieve words for immediate use.

Receptive language the ability to comprehend the spoken word, encompasses reading.

Redundancy the abundance of informational cues inherent in a message such that if parts of the message is omitted it would not distort the overall meaning of the message.

Resistance to distortion the ability to process information even though the message is distorted by noise.

Reticular activating system (RAS) a network of nuclei and neural multisynaptic pathways connecting all levels of the brainstem with the cerebral cortex, which constitutes the activating and integrating of systems to promote motivation and attention and facilitate or inhibit the process of coding, and this extends from the medulla oblongata to the thalamus in the midbrain connecting fibers to and from the cerebrum, sometimes called the *general alarm system*.

Reverberation the persistence of a sound wave as a result of multiple reflections off smooth surfaces in an enclosed space after direct sound has ceased.

Scanning the ability to survey one's storage of auditory experiences to match previous data with the present auditory experience.

Selective attention the ability to focus on a primary signal without being distracted by competing sound sources within one's environment.

Sensorineural hearing loss a hearing impairment due to dysfunction of the end organ of hearing and its auditory neural pathways.

Sequencing the organizing of a series of individual sounds in their correct order.

Signal-to-noise ratio the relationship between the intensity of a signal and noise present.

Speech discrimination a person's ability to tell whether two sounds are the same or different.

Glossary

Speech recognition the ability to recognize speech by reproducing it in some way.

Synapse a point or junction at which impulses move from one neuron to another *(neurotransmission)*.

Verbal Sequential Memory the ability to remember sounds in words and words in sentences in their proper sequential order.

Word deafness the inability of a person with normal hearing to understand what is said.

References

Allen, D. V. Modality aspect of mediation in children with normal and impaired hearing acuity. *Final Report*, Project No. 7-0837, Bureau of Education for the Handicapped, Wayne State University, Detroit, 1969.

Aoki, C., Siekevitz, P. Plasticity in brain development. *Sci. Am.,* 259, 56-64, 1988.

Barnes, S. B., Gutfreund M., Satterly, D. J. Characteristics of adult speech which predict children's language development. *J. Child Lang.*, 10:65-84, 1983.

Barr, D. F. and Carlin, T. W. *Auditory Perceptual Disorders.* Springfield, Ill: Charles C. Thomas, 1972.

Bellis, T. J. *Assessment and Management of Central Auditory Processing Disorders in the Educational Setting.* San Diego, California, <u>Singular Publishing Group</u>, 1998.

Blager, F., and Martin, H. P. Speech and language of abused children. In Martin H. P and Kempe C. H (Eds.), *The Abused Child,* Cambridge, MA: Ballinger, 1976, pp. 83-92.

Bronfenbrenner, U. *A Report on Longitudinal Evaluations of Preschool Programs, Vol. 11, is Early Intervention Effective?* US Department of Health, Education and Welfare Publication No. (OHD) 75-25, 1974.

Bryden, M. Ear preference in auditory perception. *J. Exp. Psych.*, 16, 359-360, 1963.

Burns, M. S. Access to Reading: the language to Literacy Link. A paper presented at the Learning Disabilities Association Conference. Scientific Learning Corp. University Avenue, Berkeley, CA, February, 1999.

CASLPO *State-of-the-Profession Report* (2). Toronto, Ontario, Canada, June 4, 2001, p. 3.

Cicchetti, D., and Beeghly, M. Symbolic development in maltreated youngsters: An organizational perspective. In Cicchetti D., and Beeghgly M. (Eds.), *Atypical Symbolic Development*. San Francisco, CA: Joseey-Bass, 1987, pp. 47-68.

Dirks. D. Perception of dichotic and monaural verbal material and cerebral dominance for speech. *Acta Oto-laryngology*, 58, 78-80, 1964.

Fox, L., Long, S. H., and Langlois, A. Patterns of language comprehension deficit in abused and neglected children. *J. Speech Hear. Disord.*, 53:239-244, 1988.

Friedlander, B. Z. Receptive language development in infancy: issues and problems. *Merrill-Palmer Quart*, 16:7-51, 1970.

Frisina, D. R. Some problems confronting children with deafness. *Except. Child.*, 26:94-98, 1959.

Garrison, K. C., and Force, D. G. (4th Ed.). *The Psychology of Exceptional Children*. New York: Ronald Press, 1965.

Geschwind, N. Neurological foundations of language. In Myklebust (Ed.). *Progress in learning disabilities*. New York: Grune and Stratton, 1967.

Greenwald, J. Retraining your brain. *Time Magazine*, Time Inc., July 5, 1999.

Haggard, M. P., and Hughes, E. A. Screening children's hearing: A review of the literature and implications of otitis media. London: HMSO, 1991.

Hargrove, P. M., Roetzel K., and Hoodin, R. B. Modifying the prosody of a language-impaired child. *Language Speech and Hearing Services in Schools (ASHA)*, 20, 245-258, 1989.

Hebb, D. O. *The Organization of Behavior*. New York: John Wiley & Sons, 1949.

Holtz, L. In Art of Language, the Brain Matters. *Los Angeles Times*, October, 1998.

Hughes, H. M., and DiBrezzo R. Physical and emotional abuse and motor development: A preliminary investigation. *Percept Mot Skills*, 64:469-470, 1987.

Johnson, C. J. Language and academic outcomes of children with preschool language disorders, Conference presentation: The spectrum of development disabilities XX111: Disorders of language development-stages or continuum? March 26-28, 2001.

Johnson D. L. and Myklebust, H. R. *Learning Disabilities: Educational Principles and Practices*, New York: Grune and Straton, 1971. Joint Committee on Infant Hearing, Position Statement, 1994.

Karlin, I. Speech and language handicapped children. *J. Dis. Child.,* 95:370-376, 1958.

Kimura, D. Some effects of temporal-lobe damage on auditory perception. *Can. J. of Psych.,* 15, 156-165, 1961a.

Kolata, G. Studying learning in the womb: Behavioral scientists are using established experimental methods to show that fetuses can and do learn. *Sci.,* 20:302-303, 1984.

Kodman, F. Identification of Hearing Loss by Parents and Teachers. *Maico Au diological Library Series V. 11,* p. 32, 1978.

Martmer, E. D. *The Child with a Handicap.* Springfield, IL: Charles Thomas, 1959.

McCauley R., Swisher, L. Are maltreated children at risk for speech or language impairment? An unanswered question. *J. Speech Hear. Disord.* 52:301-303, 1987.

OSLA. Speech Language Services in Ontario Schools, A working document., Toronto, Canada, March 18, 1996.

Penfield, W. and Roberts, L. *Speech and brain mechanism*, Princeton: Princeton University Press, 1959.

Pillsbury, H. C., Grose, J. H., and Hall, J. W. Otitis media with effusion in children. *Archives of Otolaryngology, Head and Neck Surgery*, 117, 718-723, 1991.

Pinheiro, M. L. Tests of central auditory function in children with learning disabilities. In Keith, R. W. (Ed.), *Central Auditory Dysfunction.* New York: Grune & Stratton, 1977.

Pinker, S. *The Language Instinct: How the Mind Creates Language.* New York: Harper Perennial, 1994.

Rauschecker, J. P., and Marler, P. Cortical plasticity and imprinting: behavior and physiological contrasts and parallels. In J. P. Rauschecker and P. Marler (Eds.), *Imprinting and Cortical Plasticity* (pp. 349-366). New York: John Wiley & Sons, 1987.

Richardson, S. O. Communication results of central auditory tests with other professionals. In Keith, R. W. (Ed.), *Central Auditory Dysfunction*, New York: Grune & Stratton, 1977.

Rips, L. J., Shoben, E. J., and Smith, E. E. Semantic distance and the verification of semantic relations. *J. Verbal Learn. Behav.*, 12:1-20, 1973.

Russell, W. and Espir, M. *Memory and Learning: A Neurologist's View.* London: Oxford University Press, 1961.

Satz, K., Achenback, E., Pattishall, and Fennell, E. Order of report, ear asymmetry and handedness in dichotic listening. *Cortex*, 1, 377-395, 1965.

Smith, E. E., Shoben, E. J. and Rips, L. J. Structures and process in semantic memory. A featural model for semantic decision. *Psychol. Rev.,* 81:214-241, 1974.

Walsh, R. N., and Greenough, W. T. (Eds.), *Environment as Therapy for Brain Dysfunction.* New York: Plenum, 1976.

Weaver, C. H., Furbee, Catherine and Everhart, R. W., Paternal occupational class and articulatory defects in children. *J. Speech and Hearing Disord.*, 25:171-175, 1960.

Suggested Reading

Bond, J. Effects of noise on the physiology and behavior of farm-raised animals. In B. L. Welch and A. S. Welch (Ed.). *Physiological Effects of Noise*, New York: Plenum Press, 1970, pp. 295-306.

Brandes, P. and Ehinger, D. The effect of early middle ear pathology on auditory perception and academic achievement. *J. Speech Hear. Disord.*, 46:301-307, 1981.

Broadbent, D. E., Effects of noise on behavior. In Harris, C. M. (Ed.), *Handbook of Noise Control*, New York: McGraw Hill Book, Chapter 10, 1957.

Cantwell, D. P., and Baker L: *Psychiatric Developmental Disorders in Children with Communication Disorders*. Washington, DC: American Psychiatric Press, 1991.

Cohen, A. Noise, effects on health, productivity and well-being. *Transactions of New York Academy of Science*, Series 11, Vol. 30, 1968.

Crow, A. *An Outline of Educational Psychology*. New Jersey: Littlefield, Adam & Co., 1968.

Fox, L., Long, S. H., Langlois, A., Patterns of language comprehension deficit in abused and neglected children. *J. Speech Hear. Disord.*, 53:239-244, 1988.

Hernandez-Peón, R., Scherrer, H., and Jouvet, M., Modification of electric activity in cochlear nucleus during attention in unanesthetized cats. *Sci.*, 123:331-332, 1956.

Hernandez-Peon, R., Reticular mechanisms of sensory control. In Rosenblith, W. A., (Ed.), *Sensory communication*. Cambridge: MIT Press, pp. 497-520, 1961.

Katz, J. and Cohen, C. F. Auditory training for children with processing disorders. *J. Childhood Comm. Disord.* Vol. 1X, 1985.

Kendel, E. R., Schwartz, J. H. and Jessell, T. M. (Eds.), *Principles of Neural Science* (3rd ed.). East Norwalk, CT: Appleton and Lange, 1991.

Kirk, S., and W. Kirk, *Psycholinguistic Learning Disabilities: Diagnosis and Remediation*. Urbana, Ill.: University of Illinois Press, 1969.

Lenneberg, E. H. *Biological foundations of language*. New York: John Wiley & Sons, 1967a.

Lenneburg, E. H. Prerequisites for language acquisition. *Proceedings of the International Conference on Oral Education of the Deaf,* 1302-1362. Washington: The Volta Review. (1967b).

Levitan, I. B. and Kaczmarek, I. K. *The Neuron: Cellular and Molecular Biology*. New York: Oxford University Press, 1997.

Mark, H. J. Psychodiagnostics in patients with suspected minimal brain dysfunction(s), appendix B, Minimum Brain Dysfunction in Children. Public Health Services Publishers. No. 2015, 1969, pp. 75-76.

Martmer, E. D. *The Child with a Handicap*. Springfield, Ill.: Charles Thomas, 1959.

McCauley R., and Swisher, L. Are maltreated children at risk for speech or language impairment? An unanswered question. *J. Speech Hear. Disord.*, 52:301-303, 1987.

Miller, I. J. and Lane, S. J. Toward a consensus in terminology in sensory integration theory and practice (Part 1): Taxonomy of neurophysiologic processes. *Sensory Integration Quarterlyl* Vol. 23 No. 1, March, 2000.

Niemeyer, W. Psychological aspects of hearing-aid fitting (Part II), *J. Audio. Tech.*, Vol. 12, No. 3, 1973.

Nober, E. H. Non-auditory effects of noise. *Maico Audiological Library Series*, Vol. X11, No. 2, 1974.

Richardson, S. O. Communication results of central auditory tests with other professionals. In Keith, R. W. (Ed.), *Central Auditory Dysfunction*, New York, Grune & Stratton, 1977.

Semel, E. *Sound, Order, Sense: A Development Program in Auditory Perception*. Chicago: Follet Educational Corporation, 1970.

Simon, D. S. (Ed.), *Communication Skills and Classroom Success: Assessment of Language Disabled Students*. College Hill Press, 1985 (available in Canada through Phonic ear, Mississauga).

Singer, J., and Hurley, R. M. Central auditory processing disorders in children. *J. Childhood Comm. Disord.* Vol. 1X, No. 1, 1985.

Warr-Leeper, G. A., Central auditory dysfunction. is anyone listening? *C.P.R.I. Profiles*, Vol. 4, No. 3, p. 14, 1983.

Waterloo County Board of Education: Special Education Services, *Central Auditory Processing: Primary, Junior, Intermediate*. Fall 19909 Revised Edition.

Whetnall, E. The young deaf child: Identification and management. In Davis, H. (Ed.), *Acta Otolaryng*, 295 (Supp.): 51, 1965.

Willeford, J. A., Audiological Evaluation of Central Auditory Disorders, *Maico Audiological Library Series*, Vol. V1, p. 2, 1969.

Willeford, J., and Burleigh, J., *Handbook of Central Auditory Processing Disorders in Children*. Grune and Stratton, Inc., 1985.

Wyatt, G., *Language, Learning and Communication Disorders in Children*. New York: Free Press, 1969.

Zigmond, N. K. and Cicci, G., Auditory Learning. In Keith E. Beery (Ed.), *Dimensions in Early Learning Series*, San Rafael, California: Dimensions, p. 21, 1968.

Additional Sources

Can J Psychiat. 32:683-687, 1987.

Child Psych. Hum. Dev., 18:191-207, 1988.

J Am Acad Child Adolesc. Psychiat 28:112-117, 19898a and 28:118-123, 1989b.

Learning Disabilities Association of Ontario, Literature Kit: Auditory-Language Learning Disabilities.

For more information on LDAO, contact their website:wwwi.ldao.on.ca

- Attention Problems or Auditory Processing?
- Central Auditory Processing Disorder
- Oral Language Problems of Adults with Learning Disabilities
- The Audiologist and Children with Learning Disabilities

Self-Evaluation Quiz

The following questions are intended to test your own understanding of the material covered. Answers to the Self-Evaluation Quiz are provided at the end of the book on pages 165 through 166. It is suggested that you use this question and answer section to review or reinforce concepts that were covered in the text for your own personal clarification and enlightenment. As a gauge to assess your understanding, each question is worth 2 percent. Here is a rough assessment of performance:

90-100   percent Outstanding

80-89   Very good grasp of concepts covered

75-79   Good grasp of concepts

70-74   Fair understanding of issues discussed

65-69   Need to review important concepts more than once

60-64   May need to reread the test for a better handle on ideas

55-59   Definitely reread the entire test with selected materials for assistance

< 55   Minimal understanding of material covered

Indicate true (T) or (F) for each statement

1.	T	F	In the process of communication development *input* precedes *output*.
2.	T	F	A child having processing difficulties manages information slowly, more slowly than his or her peers or siblings.

3.	T	F	The management team member providing valuable information regarding the social—emotional impact of the disorder and its effects on the cognitive functioning of the child is the educational audiologist.
4.	T	F	Language-impaired children may need up to 500 milliseconds to process sounds fast enough to speak or read fluently.
5.	T	F	The ability to acquire the building blocks of language is a natural phenomenon for every child.
6.	T	F	When both hemispheres of the brain are not working in perfect synchrony, a child's ability to execute certain classroom tasks simultaneously may be compromised.
7.	T	F	Subvocalization in reading should not be encouraged since it delays the development of reading skills.
8.	T	F	Every time the distance between the speaker (teacher) and the listener (child) is doubled the intensity of the speech signal is increased.
9.	T	F	A sound wave entering the ear is immediately processed by the brain for understanding.
10.	T	F	Parents do not have to be concerned if a child is not trying to talk by age one or seems insensitive to sound by this age.
11.	T	F	The ability to generalize is linked to one's ability to successfully manipulate language.
12.	T	F	Preferential seating means that the child must always be placed in the front row beside the teacher at all times during instruction.
13.	T	F	Hearing loss cannot be identified until after three months of age when the child's ear is fully functional.

14.	T	F	The unborn child still protected in its mother's womb may be capable of responding to certain sounds long before it is born.
15.	T	F	The otologist will perform a test known as an audiogram that determines the nature and extent of hearing loss.
16.	T	F	The speech-language pathologist may also be involved in the testing of the CAPD child.
17.	T	F	The brain cannot be rewired or reprogrammed once it has been fully developed.
18.	T	F	An infant developing listening skills is in a passive stage of development as he listens to sounds around him.
19.	T	F	Normal listeners do not have to hear every detail of a message to understand it.
20.	T	F	Prolonged absence of normal stimulation to the ear creates what is known as auditory sensory deprivation.
21.	T	F	When information exceeds the child's perceptual speed it will be lost.
22.	T	F	Generally speaking, the normal hearing child develops language naturally as long as he is placed in the proper environment to do so.
23.	T	F	The child with an output-organization problem does not understand well, and therefore, cannot organize an appropriate response to what he hears.
24.	T	F	The teacher must expect absolute attention at all times for the child.
25.	T	F	The distractible child is hearing too much and processes too much of what may be considered relevant information.

26.	T	F	Hearing loss is one of the most serious and least recognized disabilities in children.
27.	T	F	The teacher can experiment with the delivery system of information, varying speeds and amounts of information to determine the rate at which the child processes it.
28.	T	F	Persistent conductive hearing loss in children can affect educational performance in their formative years, resulting in long-term developmental consequences in the child's learning, social, and academic performance.
29.	T	F	This internal redundancy of the auditory system is necessary since it makes the system highly resistant to total collapse.
30.	T	F	Assistive Listening Device (ALD) is always recommended for CAPD as an educational solution to the problem.
31.	T	F	A child with decoding problems gets too much information to make sense of what he hears.
32.	T	F	Listening bridges the gap between the sounds we hear and that of attributing meaning to those sounds.
33.	T	F	The neurologist is interested in the findings of the child with central auditory disorders since they infer the developmental status of the child's central auditory nervous system that can have important implications especially for reading and language development.
34.	T	F	Environmental stimulation has little effect on the development and vitality of the human cortex.
35.	T	F	Allergies affects the child's hearing and processing from one day to the next and play a crucial role in the way he processes information from day to day.

36.	T	F	The child with an integration and separation deficiency has difficulty deciphering fine acoustic differences in sound.
37.	T	F	The recognition of nonwritten verbal information is totally dependant on the auditory system.
38.	T	F	It is the receptive phase of hearing that attributes meaning to what we hear.
39.	T	F	The alert classroom teacher should always be aware of when the child's attention is lost.
40.	T	F	Binaural separation and integration deficiency is a condition that is not crucial to everyday listening situations especially in a school environment.
41.	T	F	An expressive language deficiency is more resistant to change than a receptive language deficiency.
42.	T	F	The time at which sound becomes meaningful coincides with the ability to localize familiar sound especially the human voice.
43.	T	F	Scanning by the brain assures that storage of auditory information will always be retrieved when looking for a response to incoming stimuli.
44.	T	F	In a child with an auditory output organization deficiency, receptive language skills lags behind expressive language skills.
45.	T	F	The most constant and influential teacher of the child is the caregiver.
46.	T	F	The presence of distractions along with all other adverse elements in the learning environment at times may compete for the child's attention in the classroom.
47.	T	F	Vocabulary building improves skills for auditory closure.

48.	T	F	Reverberation is the most important factor when considering the acoustical qualities of a room.
49.	T	F	Only when the input has been properly stored will the child be able to organize an appropriate response to it.
50.	T	F	A favorable signal-to-noise ratio inevitably leads to improved speech intelligibility.
51.	T	F	The importance of active participation by caregivers is to stimulate the language processing capabilities of the child.

Author Index

Subject Index

Answers to Self-Evaluation Quiz

Question	Answer
1	T
2	T
3	F
4	T
5	F
6	T
7	F
8	F
9	F
10	F
11	T

12	F
13	F
14	T
15	F
16	T
17	F
18	F
19	T
20	T
21	T
22	T
23	F
24	F
25	F

26	T
27	T
28	T
29	T
30	F
31	F
32	T
33	T
34	F
35	T
36	F
37	F
38	F
39	T

40	T
41	F
42	T
43	F
44	F
45	T
46	T
47	T
48	T
49	T
50	T
51	T

Readers Comments

What a revelation your book has been to me! I found The Listening Child *a wonderful read for two reasons. First, I've always heard of the terms that labeled children who have disabilities in school but never really understood what they meant. Reading this book gave me great insight into the difficulties children have while learning and the importance of recognizing the signs early . . . I've gained amazing knowledge and tools to prepare me for my future career. Second, on a personal note, as a child, I struggled immensely in school and was made to feel like I was not as intelligent as my peers. Reading* Listening Child, *I was able to identify myself with the cases illustrated . . . I am on the road to self-healing and understanding. Thank you very much!* **Tammy Marcerollo**

I thoroughly enjoyed this book. It offered information from both a parent and teacher's perspective. This is exactly what I was looking for . . . I think the factor that I was least aware of was how involved the brain is in the hearing process and how complicated the actual process is. I was looking at hearing as being the primary responsibility of the actual organ—the ear. This book gives a detailed anatomy of the ear and each function the parts perform. The one expression that I found most fascinating was "the brain being wired for sound." I never thought of hearing in those terms. It is such a complicated and intricate process.

I found this book thorough and comprehensive . . . As a parent, this book has given me a more global look at my son's deficiency. As an educational assistant, this book has given me an opportunity to examine the various teaching styles that may be appropriate in my school setting . . . I would suggest that this book be a part of the teacher resource library that should be offered in every school. **Terry Wilkinson**

The Listening Child *has given me a solid foundation for understanding the mechanics of hearing (the ear), the processes by which information is interpreted in the brain (perceptive hearing), and the challenges which may occur if there is a problem in any one of these processes . . . This book has definitely peaked my interest in this area of education. It was written with a balance of scientific and technical information, practical and real life studies of children who may be experiencing listening disorders. My favorite chapter was the last "A Final Word to Teachers: Teaching Success with CAPD." I think it was full of practical advice and suggestions for reaching the child and helping each individual to learn to the best of their ability . . . I have gained a lot of valuable knowledge and have been given tools to make my work with children a success.* **Anne Stevens**

The title Why Johnny Isn't Learning: Noise and the Mind *caught my eye, and I was hooked. It was only natural that I would want to explore this further in the sequel, 'The Listening Child: What Can Go Wrong?' I found detailed information about the processes that are involved in auditory communication and how a child listens and interprets information and what happens when they are not able to distinguish sounds. I was able to find out more and in greater detail of how extensive this condition can be and its affects on children in both academic and social settings. Thank you, Dr. Prescod.* **Jessica Putnam**

Stephen Prescod's book, The Listening Child: What Can Go Wrong? *is packed full of useful information on the subject of how listening problems affect children's ability to learn. This book will be very useful in my future career as an educational assistant. For me, it will be a guideline or a reference book . . . As a parent of two young children, I am concerned with their education. I hope never to have them diagnosed with a listening disorder. I have learned that it is my responsibility as a parent to look for signs of these disorders for early prevention. If my child does have a listening disorder, I will use this book very frequently to help him.* **Melanie Mclean**

Thank you for the awareness this book has brought me and the increased patience and hope it has given me for the day-by-day support I can give to children with listening and other learning disorders. **Irene Metzger**

This was my first course since high school, and I was quite intimidated. Then I read the following paragraph found on p. 2 of this book The Listening Child: What Can Go Wrong? *The child's poor self-esteem and his subaverage academic performance are intricately interrelated and form an integral part of his overall developmental delay. Management must focus on rebuilding self-confidence from an image that has been shattered by a revolving cycle of relentless failure. I credit the presentation of the text with much of the comfort level I have achieved. I have gone over sections of this book to research on the symptoms and medical terminology. I intend to keep it close at hand as a resource when I am working in the classroom with children with listening disorders . . . It is a reliable, informative, and hope-filled guide . . . an essential addition to the library of anyone, from students to otologists, who are touched personally by a child with listening disorders.* **Ruth Sproule**

When I read your book, I felt that it answered some of the questions that nobody else could answer. Reading your book made me look at each child as an individual. **Lisa Hoegy**

From the point of view of a former high school teacher, I have found this book very enlightening for various reasons. First, it has made me aware of how incredibly complex the delicate workings of the ear and brain are, and I now regard the sense of hearing with new respect rather than simply taking it for granted. Second, I have gained insight into the problems experienced by some of my former pupils. I found the case history studies in chapters 5-7 particularly interesting as I was able to relate some of the experiences of the children whose listening and resulting learning problems were analyzed in these chapters. I think that I could have been more effective as a teacher in dealing with children with impaired listening skills, had I read this book as part of my training. **Fenella Laband**

Overall, this book is very informative, well laid out, and relatively easy to understand. It provides a good basic understanding of the listening disorders and is an excellent resource . . . The final chapter: "A Final Word to Teachers" is very beneficial to anyone working in the classroom. **Cheryl Weishar**

I find Dr. Prescod's explanations complete and convincing, especially the part dealing with "How children with listening problems of children. The distinction between merely hearing and truly listening is very helpful. What I like best about this book is its positive emphasis on the possibility of improvement where listening problems exist. It shines with hope! *There is in it also, I think, a delight in the wonderful way we humans are made. The brain is a most amazing thing! I like too the way our individuality as learners is recognized, appreciated, and allowed for in the suggested management of any difficulties a specific learner might have. There is a respect for each child . . . Thank you, Dr. Prescond, for teaching us so much about the listening child and not only about what goes wrong but also about what can be set right.* **Arvilla Sigma**

In all, I found your book to be a great resource that I am sure to refer to and lend to educators in the future. It is a book that I would recommend to anyone involved with a child who has listening, processing, and attention problems. **Francine Flynn**

The book The Listening Child: What Can Go Wrong? *gives a great overview of the anatomy of the ear and the brain, thus providing a basic knowledge base on how normal hearing, listening, and processing takes place. I found this section of the book very helpful in visualizing the process (of listening and interpreting) as it happens. This is necessary to understand the information that follows in the rest of the book.* **Tracy Pitcher**

Delving into the mind of the "challenged" child is a very complex and fascinating topic. The precise and detailed information described about how hearing and processing can have such a profound outcome on learning is remarkable. This is a very useful book for both parents and educators . . . *Certain indicators of behaviors are warnings of serious hearing or processing malfunctions and serve to bring about some understanding and compassion. The caregiver or the educator in turn can put a child on the road to getting proper medical attention and help.* **Sandra Kropf**

This book contains a lot of valuable information, and I feel teachers should be made to read it. **Linda Ghent**

I found reading The Listening Child like putting together a jigsaw puzzle. When all the pieces are together, you are able to see the big picture. Overall, I found the text to be very interesting and informative. **Shiela Paton**

I found that chapter 4 was the most inspiring for me with its details of how we process information . . . I never knew so much had to happen in order for us to hear. It is something that I obviously haven't appreciated and will never take for granted again. **Linda Cabral**

This book will be a useful resource in my classroom. I enjoyed the book and was captivated with each chapter. I emphasize that we will see children with listening disorders in a different light because of this book by Dr. Stephen Prescod. **Normajean Diefenbaker**